IMAGES
of America

THE LEGACY OF NURSING AT ALBANY MEDICAL CENTER

Mary D. French and Elsie L. Whiting

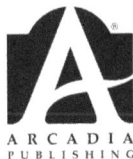

ARCADIA
PUBLISHING

Published by Arcadia Publishing
Charleston, South Carolina

Library of Congress Catalog Card Number: 2003113358

For all general information, contact Arcadia Publishing:
Telephone 843-853-2070
Fax 843-853-0044
E-mail sales@arcadiapublishing.com
For customer service and orders:
Toll-free 1-888-313-2665

Visit us on the Internet at www.arcadiapublishing.com

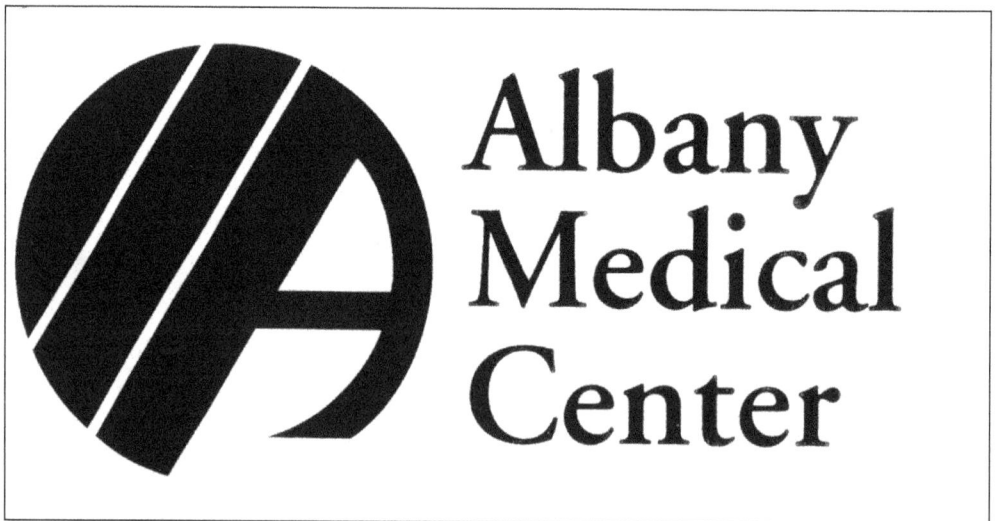

THE ALBANY MEDIAL CENTER LOGO. Just as the pillars have become a symbol representing Albany Medical Center (AMC), so has the "flying A," which was introduced in 1982. The noted logo was created when Albany Medical College and Albany Medical Center Hospital (AMCH) joined under one board of governors. The "flying A" really soars when helicopters of the area's only dedicated air medical transport program are in the skies or landing on the heliport on the D building's roof.

CONTENTS

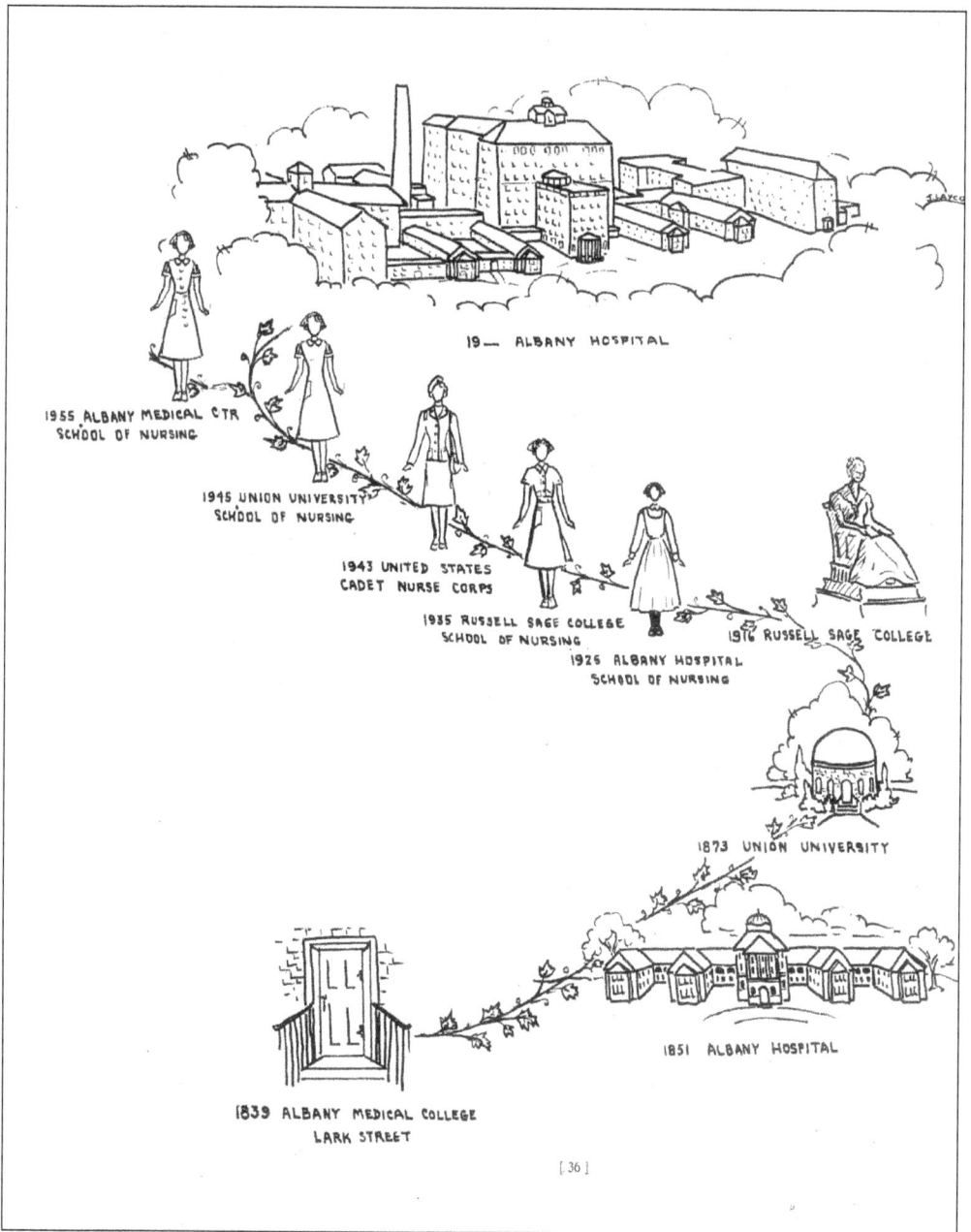

NURSING TIMELINE HIGHLIGHTS. Editorial license was taken to update and include Albany Medical Center School of Nursing in the timeline that Jeanne Laycock created for her U.S. Cadet Nurse Corps yearbook, *Tres Anni,* for the Class of 1947, section 2. Albany Hospital (AH) opened in 1849 and was formally dedicated in 1851. Albany Hospital Training School for Nurses (AHTSN) began in 1897, and the school pin changed in 1925. The open date for Albany Hospital (now Albany Medical Center Hospital) represents the ongoing changes that occur to maintain its state-of-the-art status in care, research, and education.

6

INTRODUCTION

Few cities in America have as rich a tradition in nursing education as Albany. During the past century, there were many nursing schools affiliated with what is now known as Albany Medical Center. This book is an attempt to build upon earlier efforts and to familiarize all interested with this fascinating history of nursing education and practice here, in New York's capital.

It is appropriate to begin by saluting Louise Denison, R.N., Class of 1928, who first began compiling this history. Her countless hours of research and copious notes on salient information "entailed voluminous reading, many personal interviews and an earnest attempt to piece together fragments of pertinent data into a meaningful whole." The notes were preserved by the Albany Medical Center Schools of Nursing Alumni Association. Her presence is with us in these excerpts from her manuscript:

> Albany, and its surrounding area can be justly proud of the schools of nursing that have been associated with the Albany Hospital, later known as the Albany Medical Center. These schools existed to educate area nurses beginning in 1897 and continuing until 1989 when each graduate of the last class completed their basic nursing preparation. The four schools within the Alumni Association are: the Albany Hospital Training School for Nurses, (AHTSN) 1897-1937; the U.S. Cadet Nurse Corps associated with Russell Sage College School of Nursing (RSCSN) and Albany Hospital, which included a nationwide, emergency, wartime program, 1942-1947; the Union University School of Nursing, (UUSN) a division of the Albany Medical College, 1945-1957 and the Albany Medical Center School of Nursing, (AMCSN) 1955-1989.
>
> These years were marked by countless discoveries in science, technology and media. Think of the strides in nursing education alone! As Marie Treutler, second Director of the last of the four schools, said so succinctly, "From turpentine stupes we have come to organ transplants and heart-lung machines, and from flaxseed poultices to the miracles of antibiotics and hemodialysis." She also might have added, "from the use of emetics and purges to the use of tranquilizers and specific specialized medications to rid a patient of convulsions."
>
> It is hoped you will experience some of the hopes, anxieties, and the last-minute confusions attending the opening of our first school of nursing in 1897. The school sprang into being within a span of six short months, between the issuance of Dr. Albert Vander Veer's letter of June 1, 1896, and the opening of the school the following January, in 1897. Comprehension of this is truly mind-boggling!
>
> Consider also the diversity of opinions held regarding entry of the United States into the hostilities of World War I as well as the haste necessary and problems met in readying Base Hospital #33 for service. The extreme shortage of nurses was intensified by the catastrophic effect of the influenza epidemic which occurred during both World Wars. And finally, imagine the heartaches and the joys felt by participants at our last graduation festivities in 1989, and the pathos attending the demolition of the Nurses' Residence. What a history it has been!

The Alumni Association has been tireless in its efforts to preserve the schools' histories as seen in the exhibits throughout the Main 4 corridors of AMCH, featuring caps from the various nursing schools, graduation class photographs, a nurse doll collection, and other salient artifacts. Additionally, the association produced the video *Alumni Remembrances 1897–1989*, which captured valuable oral history from many nursing school graduates. Installed in May 2003, the nursing history exhibit in the Pillars Lobby was the result of the combined efforts of the Albany Medical Center Foundation and hospital nursing staff, along with alumni, who worked together to compile a historical timeline of nursing at Albany Medical Center.

Journey with us through chapter 1, where the beginnings not only of the first school but also of the modern nursing were founded on Florence Nightingale's principles. Having weathered the flu epidemic and World War I, over 1,000 nurses had graduated when AHTSN closed in 1937.

Chapter 2 covers the evolution of nursing education and practice from the nurse as a handmaiden to nursing as a profession. The years between 1934 and 1989 show a time of struggle for the recognition of nursing as a profession, with the debate of education centered on whether the diploma program should remain under the aegis of hospital governance or move under the aegis of a college that would grant associate or baccalaureate degrees. During this period, Russell Sage College was affiliated with Albany Hospital and Albany Medical College for clinical instruction and practice from 1934 to 1944. A further connection existed from 1942 to 1947, when the U.S. Cadet Nurse Corps at Russell Sage College was affiliated with Albany Hospital. Beginning in 1945, Union University School of Nursing as a school of Union University and as a division of Albany Medical College offered the opportunity to earn a nursing diploma or, with 60 additional liberal arts college credits, to be awarded a baccalaureate degree in nursing. The School of Nursing at Russell Sage College, as well as the division of School Nurse-Teacher Education at Plattsburgh State Teachers College, affiliated with Union University's nursing program. Because this program was not attracting a sufficient number of nursing students, the Albany Medical Center School of Nursing was founded in 1955 as a diploma program under Albany Hospital's board of governors. This school offered the same curriculum as Union University. Enrollment was at its peak in 1975, when a total of 173 nursing students were admitted to the spring and fall classes. Over the years, as the emphasis of nursing education progressed to the collegiate settings, diploma programs declined in number. The closure of Albany Medical Center School of Nursing occurred in 1989. Pathos was felt when the nurses' residence was demolished.

Chapter 3 features the strides of increased specialization and the evolution of nursing practice into the 21st century. The spirit of nursing lives on at Albany Medical Center. The D Wing now stands where the nurses' residence once stood and offers state-of-the-art care, with many of the nurses credentialed to deliver increasingly complex care to patients in specialized units. Most have made a commitment to lifelong nursing education as the demands require.

The Alumni Association, along with coauthors Mary D. French, R.N., and Elsie L. Whiting, R.N., is much appreciative of the abundant number and variety of photographs and images available for use in this publication, from the Albany Medical Center archives and the public-relations department as well as from members and friends of the Alumni Association and cited materials. From this excellent selection, they invite you to enjoy an exciting saga of student days of learning, caring, playing, and working, featuring the persons whose contributions made it all possible and the events of the day that impacted the nursing profession so strongly.

One

THE BEGINNINGS

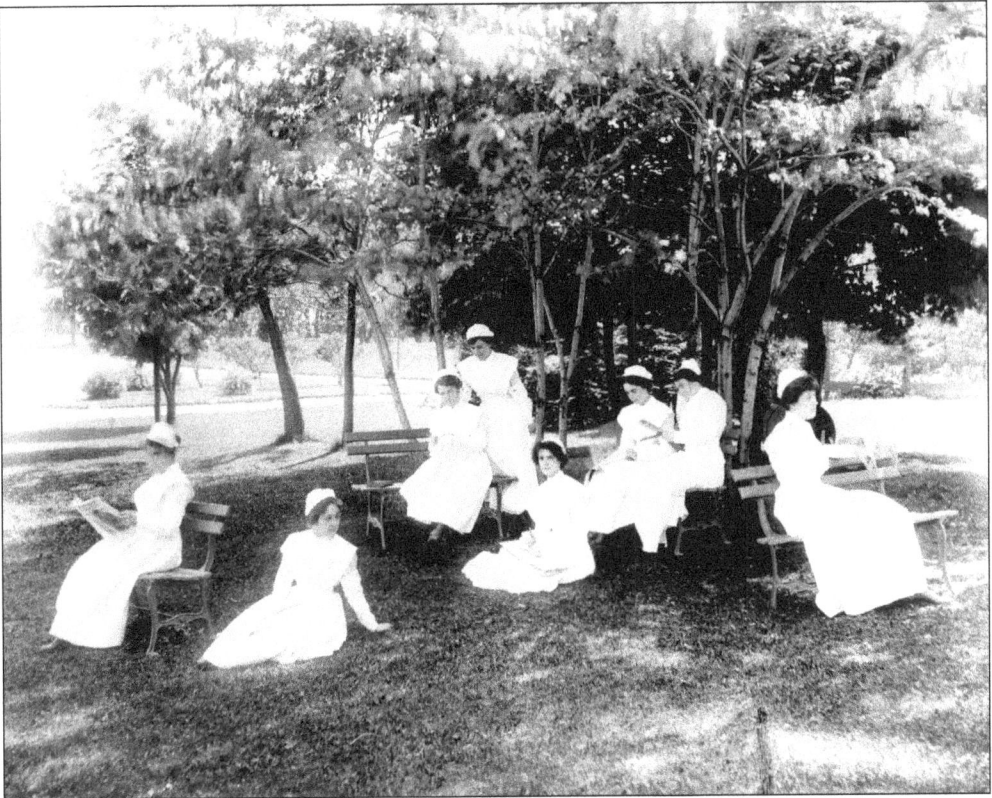

BEHIND THIS SCENE, C. 1900. These nurses look relaxed and at home on the spacious lawn at the New Scotland Avenue site of Albany Hospital, which opened in 1899. They would know that Albany Medical College was established in 1839 and that Albany Hospital first opened in 1849 at Dove Street and Lydius Street (now Madison Avenue). In 1854, the hospital moved to more adequate quarters at the corner of Eagle and Howard Streets, a site that was once home to a city jail. Perhaps these young nurses lived in Human Hall next door to the hospital. Some would share stories of what nursing was like before the training school was established and liken it to care given by the Charles Dickens character Sairey Gamp in *Martin Chuzzlewit*, who depicted the lowest in nursing. Those early periods of care for the sick cried out for improvement. The beginnings of recorded history of nursing's legacy at Albany Hospital starts with its first appearance in the board of governors' minutes and continues through the last graduate of the Albany Hospital Training School for Nurses in 1937.

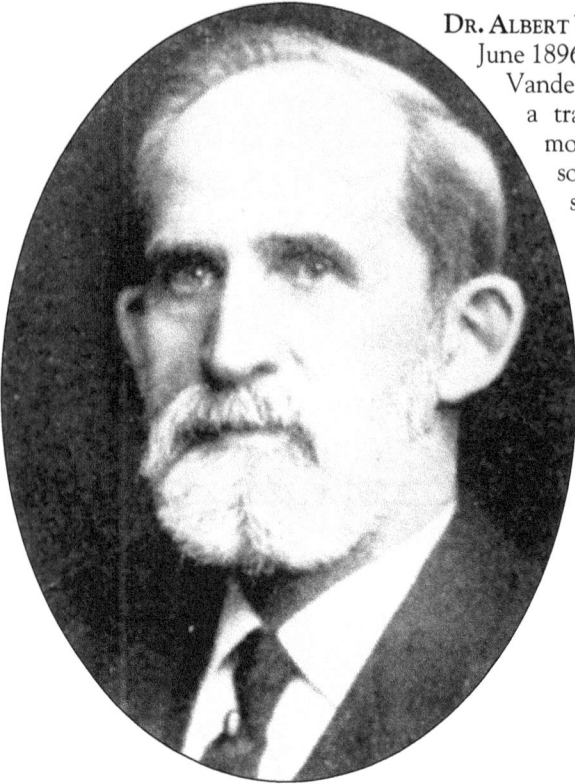

DR. ALBERT VANDER VEER. In 1893 and then again in June 1896, board of governors member Dr. Albert Vander Veer advocated the establishment of a training school for nurses. Within six months of his 1896 inquiry, the funds were solicited and support was rallied. The school was opened in January 1897. His understanding of nursing standards and acquaintance with medical and nursing leaders locally and abroad served the school well from its inception into the 1920s.

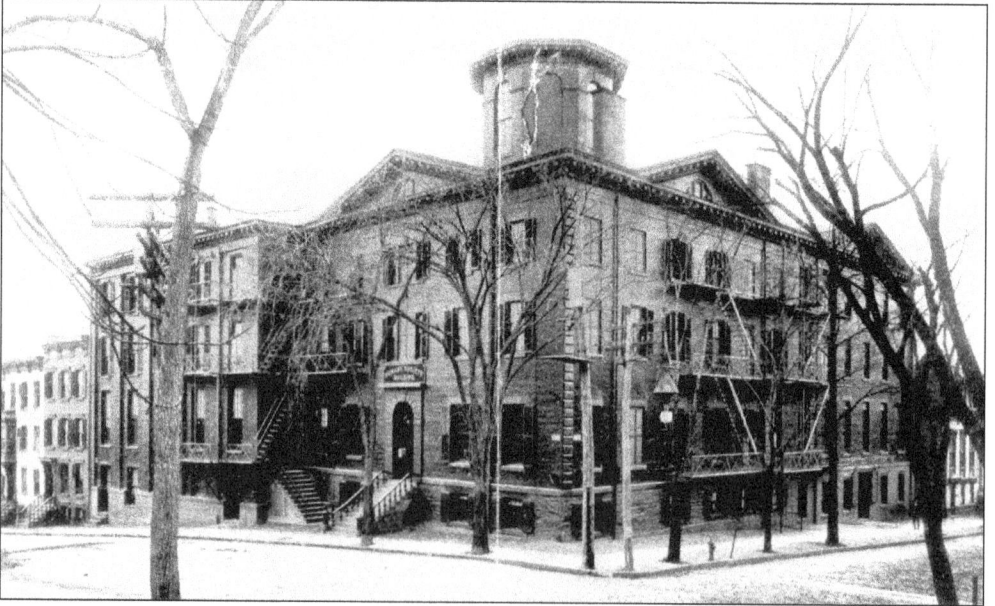

THE HOWARD STREET HOUSE. The house at 64 Howard Street, located next to the hospital and referred to as Human Hall, provided board for up to 25 nurses and pupils of the training school. In February 1897, the training school officers requested that it be repaired, and the board of governors agreed to provide the house rent-free for a year, providing that the school made its own repairs.

10

NUMBER OF PATIENTS CARED FOR IN HOSPITAL.

From March 1, 1899, to March 1, 1900.

In Hospital, March 1, 1899	93	Discharged recovered	955
Admitted during the year	1,649	Discharged improved	443
		Discharged unimproved	86
		Died	131
		In Hospital, March 1, 1900	127
Total number treated	1,742		1,742

Average number of patients each day for March, April and May quarter................................. 92$\frac{44}{91}$
Average number of patients each day for June, July and August quarter....... .... 71$\frac{58}{92}$
Average number of patients each day for September, October and November quarter................ ...... 103$\frac{53}{91}$
Average number of patients each day for December, January and February quarter................................. 124$\frac{44}{90}$
Daily average for the year... 97$\frac{110}{865}$
Number of days' treatment of patient.. 34,540
Number of days of charity work for which the city pays at the rate of $4 per week 13,125
Number of days of charity work for which no remuneration was received.............................. 306

OUT-DOOR DEPARTMENT.

Number of treatments received by patients from March 1, 1899, to March 1, 1900...... { Males................ 3,335 / Females............. 3,662 } 6,997
Number of prescriptions made up and given away to needy patients.. 5,901

A HOSPITAL REPORT, 1899–1900. Included in this hospital report are the members of the board of managers and the patronesses. Often referred to as "lady managers," the hospital board of governors gave them authority in December 1896 "to arrange with the Training School that it provide all nursing necessary for the hospital and in consideration thereof, that there be paid to it $420 per month and the use of the house at 64 Howard St." The Out-Door Department was the dispensary, or outpatient department.

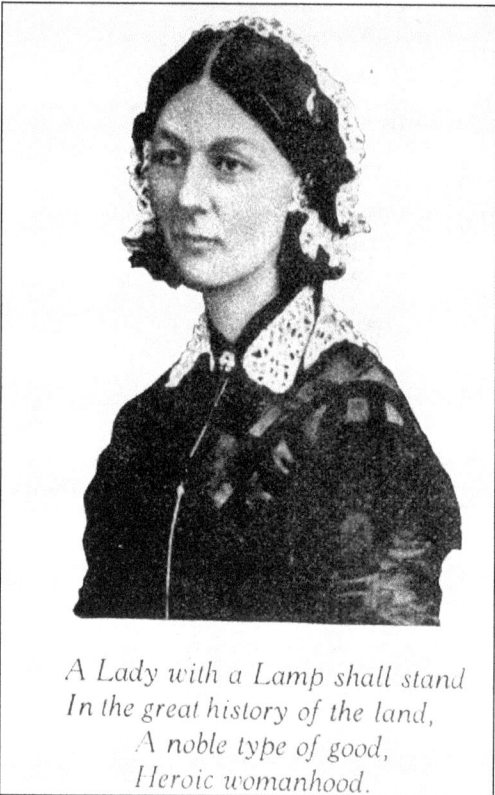

*A Lady with a Lamp shall stand
In the great history of the land,
A noble type of good,
Heroic womanhood.*

FLORENCE NIGHTINGALE. Known as the founder of modern nursing, Florence Nightingale was also called "the Soldier's Friend." During the Crimean War, she advocated that soldiers be provided fresh air, warmth, cleanliness, and a good diet, which decreased the mortality rate dramatically. The lamp she carried making rounds became the symbol representing day and night nursing service. The principles upon which she founded the Nightingale Training School for Nurses at St. Thomas's Hospital in London became the foundation of nursing schools worldwide.

THE FLORENCE NIGHTINGALE PLEDGE. Florence Nightingale is further memorialized by the pledge bearing her name, which exemplifies her professional lifestyle and which is recited by nurses at their graduation ceremonies. This custom began in 1893 and continues to the present.

I solemnly pledge myself before God and in the presence of this assembly to pass my life in purity and to practice my profession faithfully. I will abstain from whatever is deleterious and mischievous and will not take or knowingly administer any harmful drug. I will do all in my power to maintain and elevate the standard of my profession and will hold in confidence all personal matters committed to my keeping and all family affairs coming to my knowledge in the practice of my calling. With loyalty will I endeavor to aid the physician in his work and devote myself to the welfare of those committed to my care.

THE FLORENCE NIGHTINGALE PLEDGE

EMILY MACDONNELL. Emily MacDonnell (spelled McDonnell in some records) was a Johns Hopkins graduate and trained under the prestigious nurse educator Isabel Hampton Robb. In 1896, she became the first director of the newly organized nursing school. Using her strong educational background, she established entrance requirements, policies, and curriculum. A charter member of the New York State Nurses' Association, she served the school until 1905, and 109 nurses graduated under her directorship.

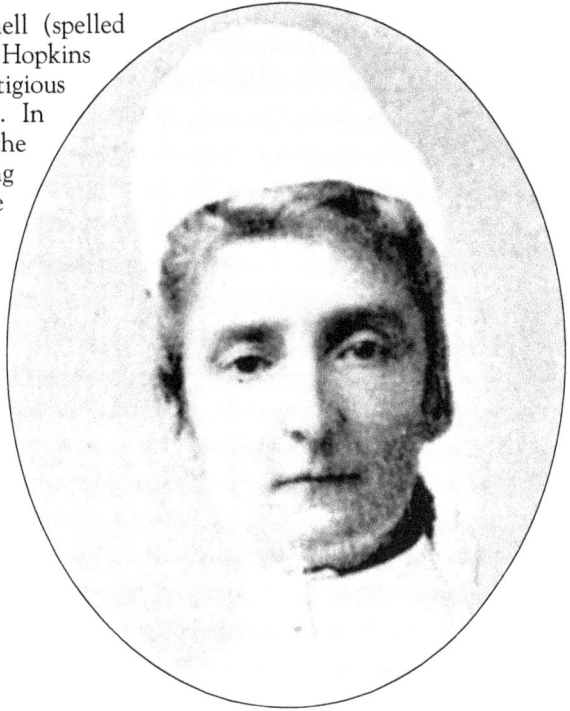

AN AGREEMENT SIGNED BY MEMBERS OF THE FIRST CLASS. Mrs. William Learned, president of the training school's board of managers, reported, "We began our work in December 1896 with three pupils who had previously been employed in the Hospital and given credit for one year of training. During 1897 we were from time to time reinforced by probationers. Though they came in slowly, by November of that year at our first annual meeting, our school numbered 19 pupils."

Employees Ticket

FOR THE
❧❧ CIRCUS ❧❧
FOR THE BENEFIT OF THE
Albany Hospital Training School for Nurses.

JUNE 22, 23, 24, 1903.

No. 89

Name...

A CIRCUS BENEFITS THE NURSING SCHOOL. A three-day circus was held for the benefit of the AHTSN from June 22 to June 24, 1903. A flyer sent by the lady managers with tickets to be purchased stated, "Albany's most prominent citizens have volunteered their services and their efforts will be supplemented by the very best professional talent obtainable in the circus line."

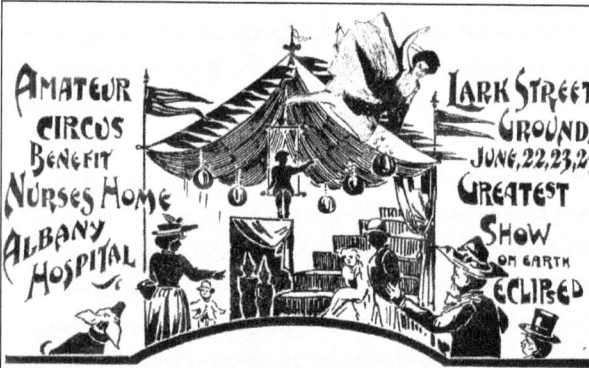

THE AMATEUR CIRCUS. In this advertisement, the circus claims to have outdone Barnum and Bailey.

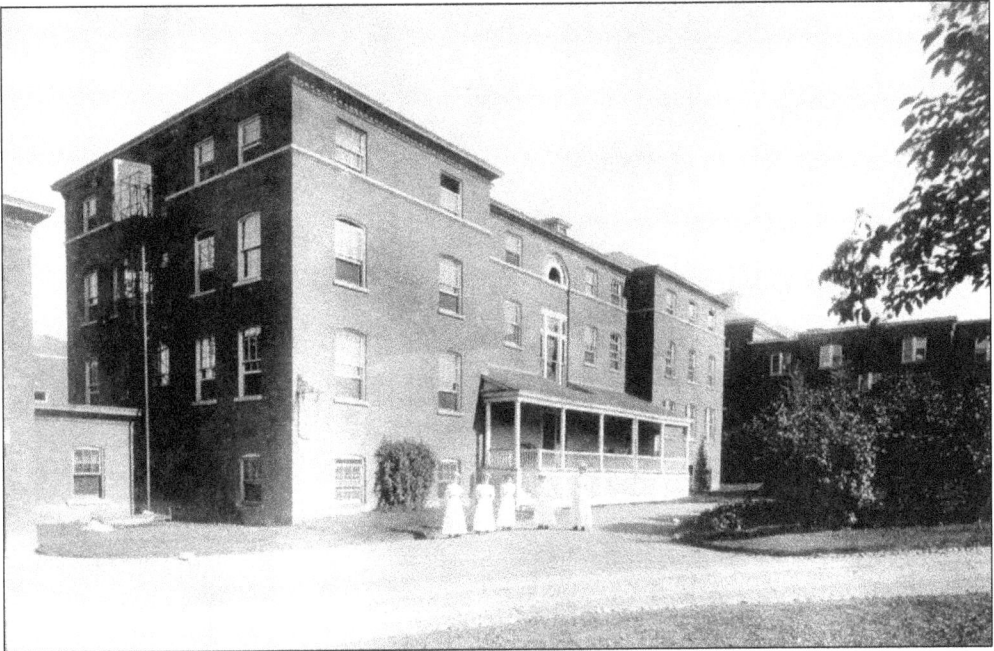

THE FIRST NURSES' RESIDENCE AT NEW SCOTLAND AVENUE. In this view, nurses stand outside their residence, located directly behind Pavilion B. By 1904, the overflow was housed in the upper story of the ambulance horse stable. In 1912, the board of governors stated that it was wise to take action to erect a new nurses' home, since 112 nurses were being educated and housed in a building originally intended for 60 nurses. Note the fire escape pole.

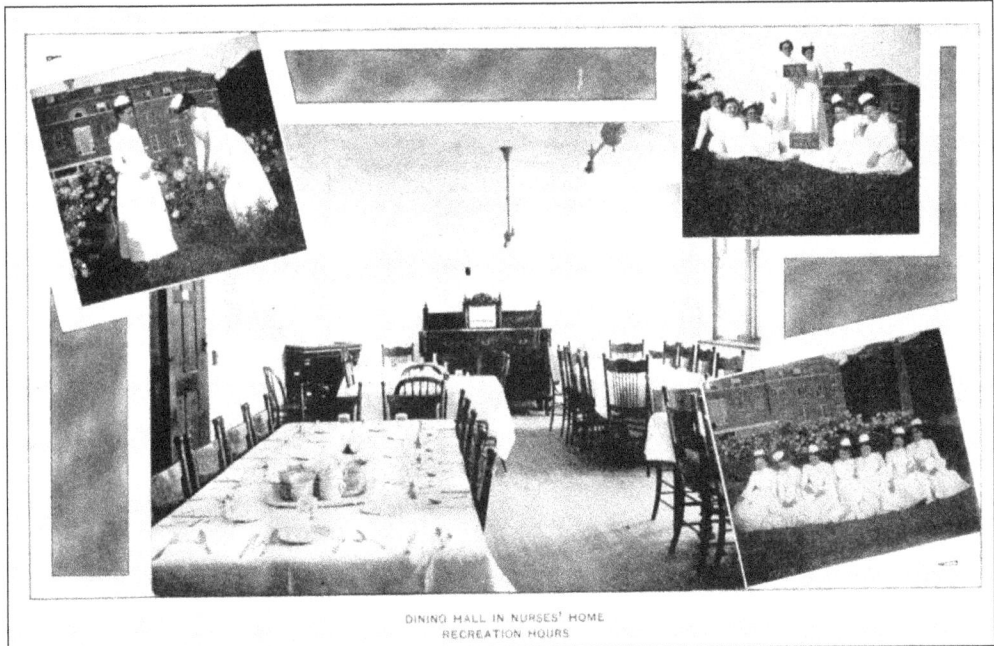

DINING HALL IN NURSES' HOME
RECREATION HOURS

THE DINING HALL IN THE NURSES' HOME AND THE COLLAGE OF RECREATION. Today's pupils might think eating in this dining room would be acceptable for a holiday dinner. Recreation never looked like this.

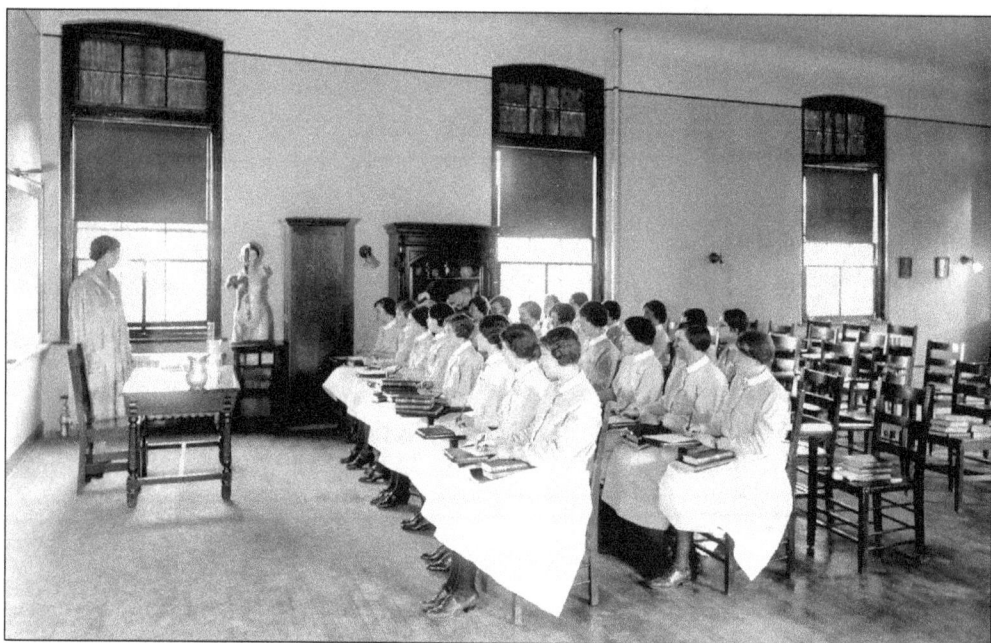

A Classroom. Pencils are poised and the pupils' attention is rapt as the lecture is given. Each is in proper uniform with every hair up off the collar. Hours for duty, including classes, were 7:00 a.m. to 7:00 p.m. days and 7:00 p.m. to 7:00 a.m. nights. Pupils were excused from duty three hours every Sunday, allowed one afternoon off each week, and allowed two hours daily for open-air exercises, study, and rest.

COURSE OF LECTURES TO NURSES

First Year

ANATOMY—Joseph D. Craig, M. D.
PHYSIOLOGY—Geo. Blumer, M. D.
HYGIENE—Willis G. Tucker, M. D.
BACTERIOLOGY—George Blumer, M. D.
OBSERVATION OF SYMPTOMS—
MATERIA MEDICA—Howard Van Rensselaer, M. D.
CIRCULATORY AND EXCRETORY SYSTEMS—Andrew MacFarlane, M. D.

Second Year

GENERAL INFECTIOUS DISEASES—Henry Hun, M. D.
SURGERY—Willis Goss Macdonald, M. D.
LUNGS—Samuel Baldwin Ward, M. D.
GYNECOLOGY—Albert VanderVeer, M. D.
OBSTETRICS—James Peter Boyd, M. D.
FRACTURES AND DISLOCATIONS—William Hailes, M. D.
INSANITY AND NERVOUS DISEASES—J. Montgomery Mosher, M. D.

Third Year

CARE OF INFANTS—James P. Boyd, M. D.
DIETETICS—J. Montgomery Mosher, M. D.
SURGICAL DISEASES OF CHILDREN—Samuel R. Morrow, M. D.
ELECTRO THERAPEUTICS—Ezra A. Bartlett, M. D.
DISEASES OF THE THROAT AND NOSE—Arthur G. Root, M. D.
DISEASES OF THE EYE AND EAR—Cyrus S. Merrill, M. D.
SKIN DISEASES—Frederic C. Curtis, M. D.
MASSAGE—Spencer L. Dawes, M. D.

The Course of Lectures to Nurses. It is interesting to note that in the earliest years of the school, courses were taught entirely by doctors. Later, catalogs began to list courses taught by nurses. A thorough curriculum was presented.

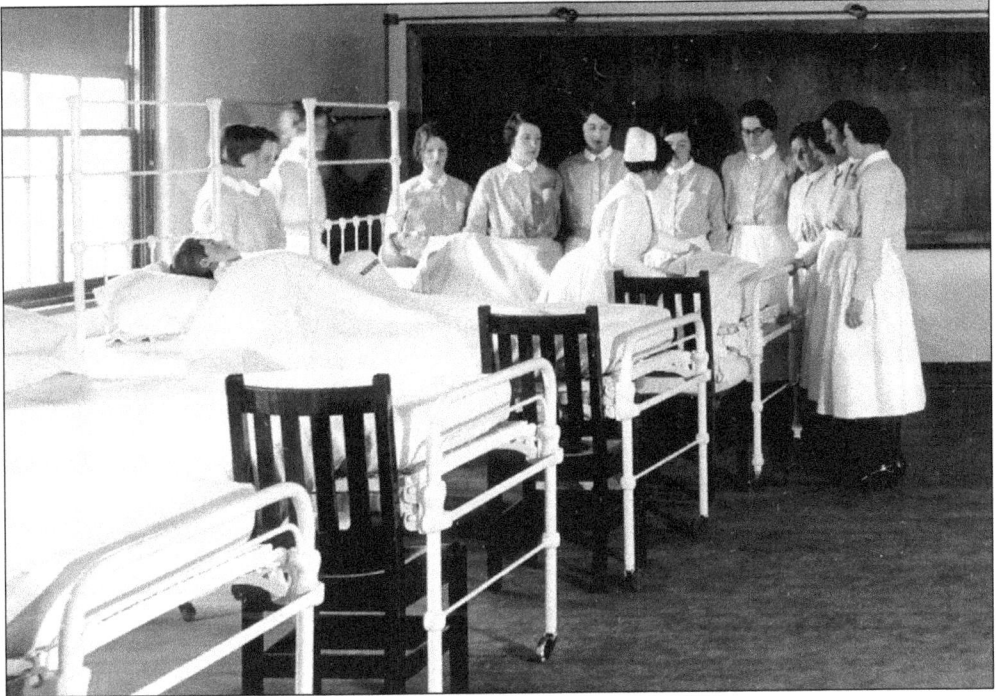

THE NURSING ARTS PRACTICE. Procedures for patient care were taught by faculty, and students were required to demonstrate their newly acquired skills. The mannequin used for practice was always named Mrs. Chase.

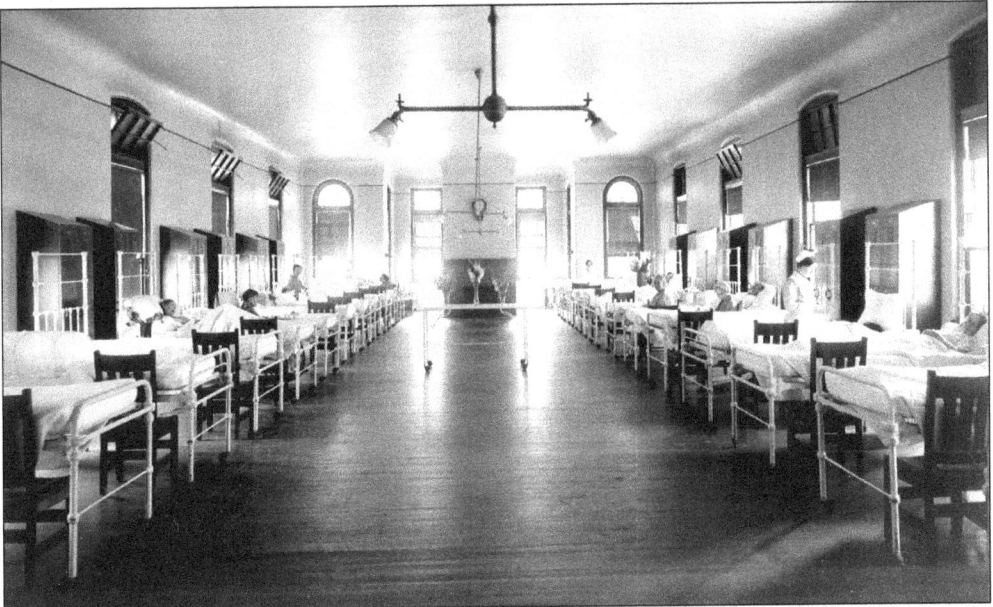

A SURGICAL WARD FOR WOMEN. The new hospital was built using the pavilion plan, which was designed to allow for fresh air and sunshine. There was a fireplace at the end of the large open room. Space between beds was at a premium, with no visible means for privacy. In addition to patient care, nurses might also be responsible for mopping floors, bringing in scuttles of coal, and washing windows once a week.

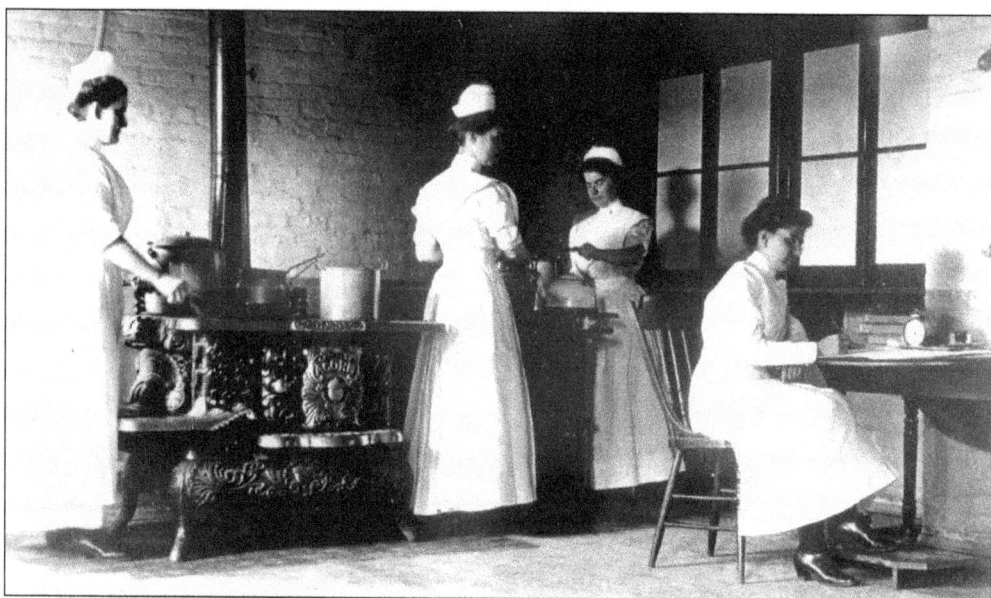

FOOD PREPARATION. Preparation of regular meals as well as special diets was a nursing duty. In 1902, the basement of the nurses' home had "an admirably arranged diet kitchen with every equipment and with a well contrived storeroom. The salary of a diet mistress was also paid."

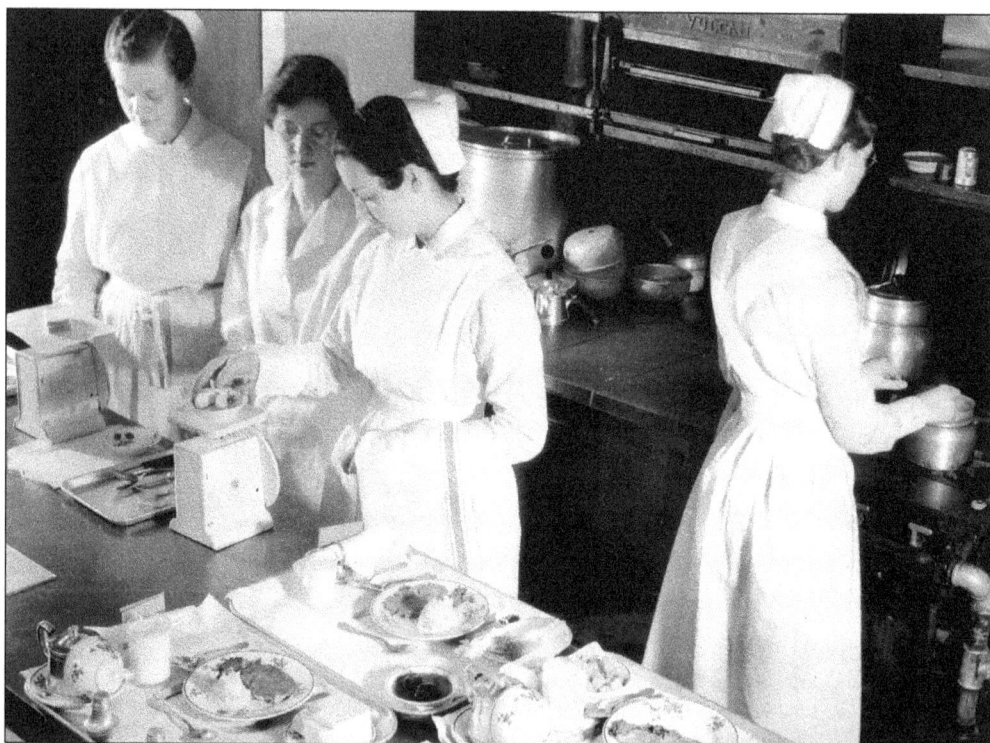

SPECIAL DIETS BEING WEIGHED. Household scales measured the correct amount of the selected food that was served on chinaware. Temperature control and cross-contamination were challenging due to the use of open trays.

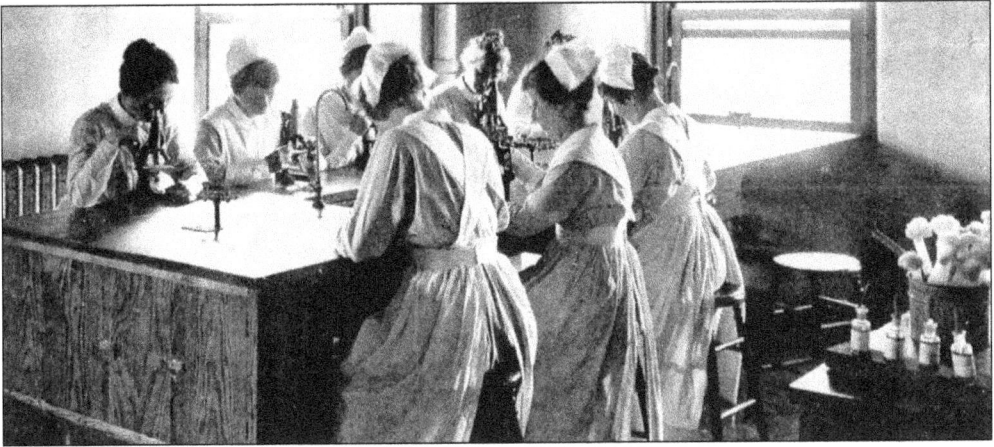

THE PATHOLOGY LABORATORY. Working in laboratories to better understand causes of illness was part of the nurses' training. In this photograph, students view slides under the microscope as part of their bacteriology course.

THE AMERICAN SOCIETY OF SUPERINTENDENTS OF TRAINING SCHOOLS FOR NURSES MEETING, 1908. Founded in 1893, this society changed its name in 1912 to the National League of Nursing Education. Also in 1912, the American Nurses' Association (ANA), the professional organization for registered professional nurses, was established as an outgrowth of the Nurses' Associated Alumnae, which began in 1896. The National Association of Colored Graduate Nurses, founded in 1908, became part of the ANA in 1951.

1908

Programme

The
Fourteenth Annual Meeting

of the

American Society

of

Superintendents of Training
Schools for Nurses.

Cincinnati, Ohio.
April 22nd, 23rd, and 24th.

Sinton Hotel.

FRIDAY, APRIL 24TH.

TEN A. M.

PAPERS.

The Nursing of Children.
SISTER AMY, S. S. M.,
The Children's Hospital, Boston, Mass.

Nursing in Diseases of the Eye and Ear,
MISS EUGENIA D. AYERS,
Manhattan Eye, Ear and Throat Hospital, New York.

A New Field—The Nurse's Opportunity in Factory Work, with a Brief Outline of Medico-Nursing Relief Work in the Westinghouse Lamp Factory,
DR. LUCY A. BANNISTER.

Introduction of President-Elect.

Adjournment.

TWO-THIRTY-FIVE P. M.

Reception to Visiting Superintendents by Woman's Club, Domestic Science Department, Mrs. J. C. Monfort, Chairman.

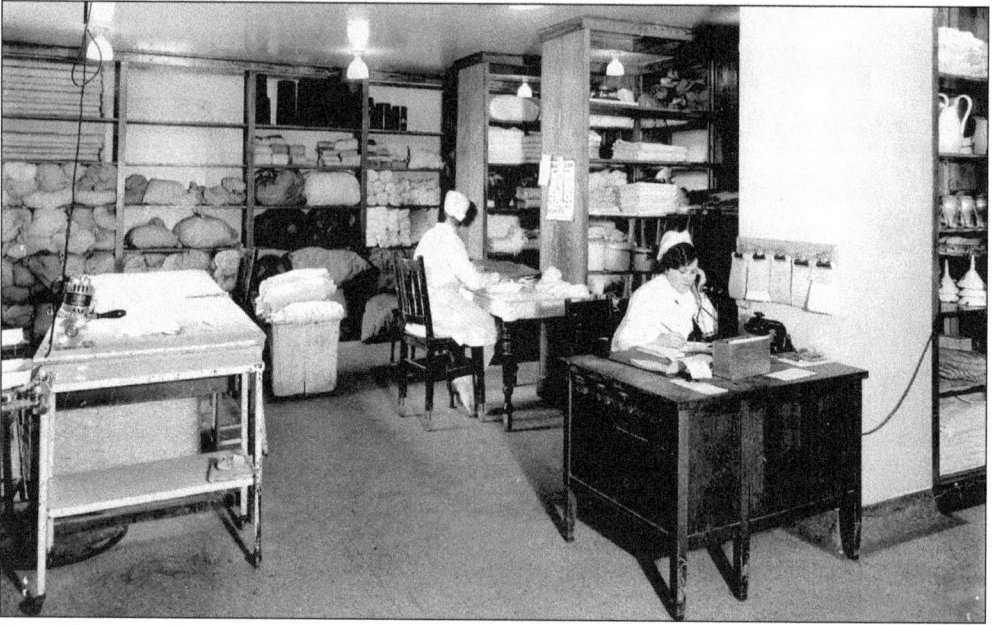

THE CONTROL STATION AND CENTRAL SUPPLY. For many years, obtaining and preparing supplies for use and filling the requests for them, as well as cleansing returned equipment, were nursing responsibilities.

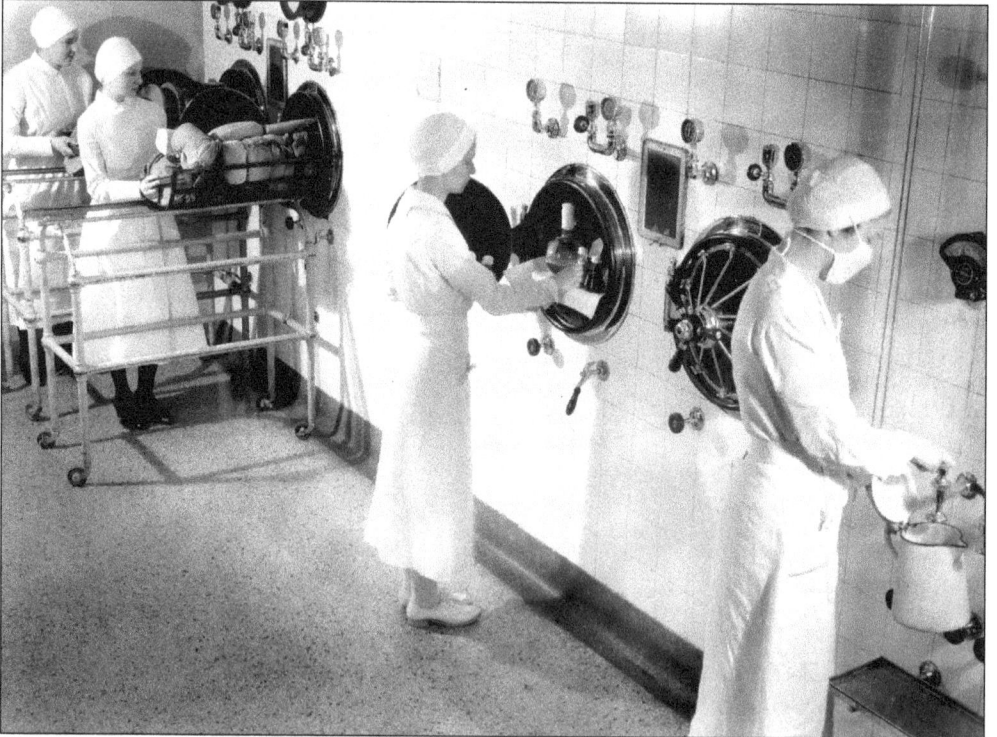

AUTOCLAVING SUPPLIES. After reusable equipment was cleaned, it had to be autoclaved and rendered sterile for reuse. Sterile packs for specific procedures were made up for operating room and ward use.

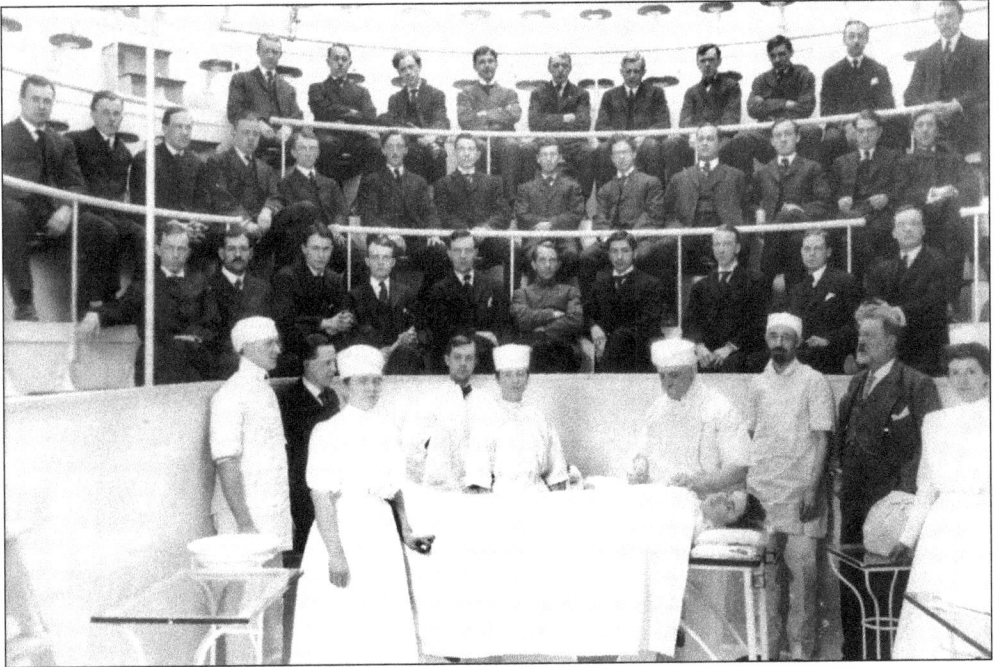

AN AMPHITHEATER DEMONSTRATION. The old-time version of closed-circuit television was a procedural demonstration given by a team of doctors and nurses in the amphitheater.

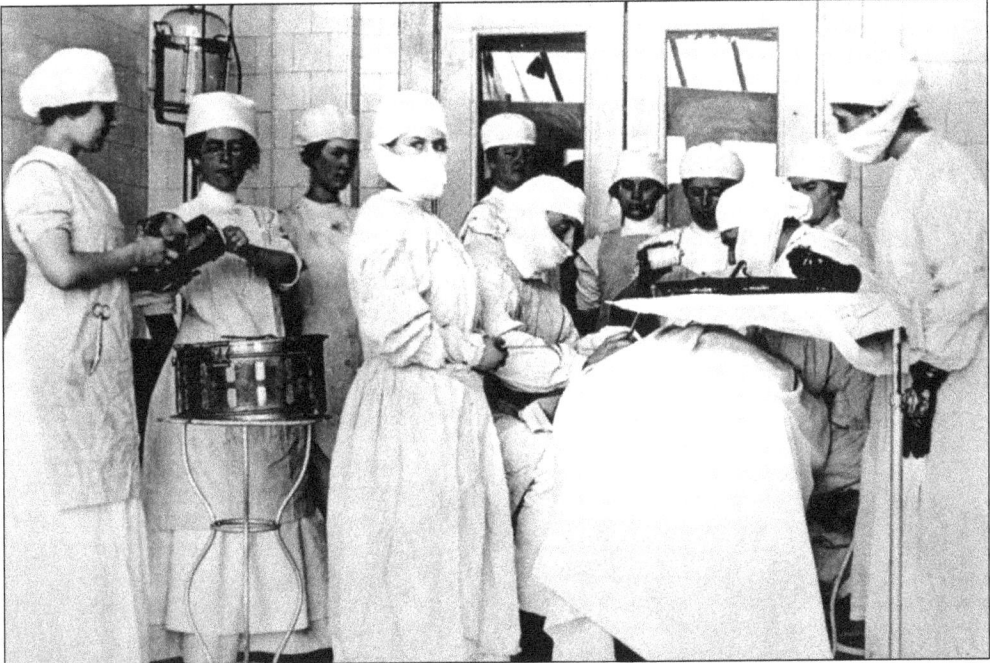

THE OPERATING ROOM. Masks appear here as gauze wraps that cover the nose of one surgeon but not of the other. This picture, dated before 1910, shows that gloves were not used by all members of the surgical team. By today's standards, the nurse with the dark gloves would be reprimanded, as her hand is below the sterile field. Hand washing and the wearing of gloves and hairnets were first practiced in operating rooms in 1891.

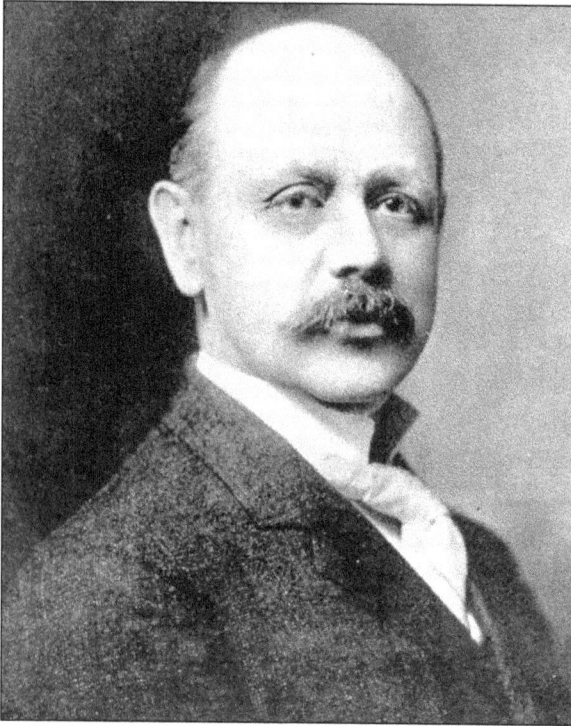

DR. JESSE MONTGOMERY MOSHER. The mentally ill were often either detained in jails or committed to asylums. Dr. Jesse Montgomery Mosher advocated that Albany County erect a ward so patients with nervous disorders could receive care available at an ordinary hospital. In 1902, Pavilion F opened with a male ward and a female ward. The first of its kind in the world, it is the oldest continuously operating psychiatric facility in a general hospital.

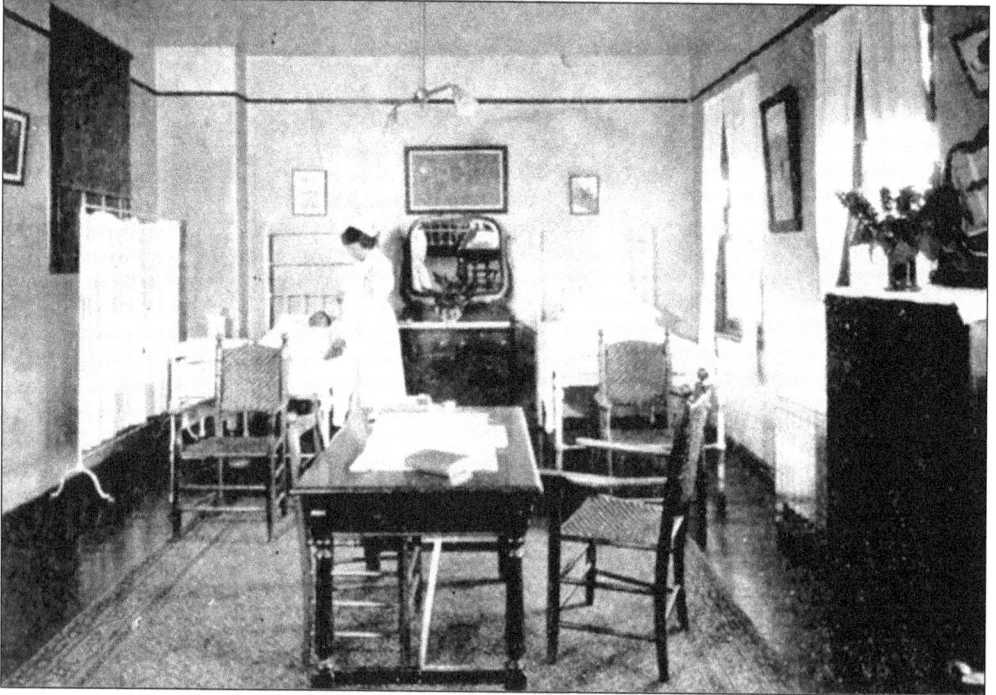

A PATIENT'S ROOM. The furnishings of this two-bed room epitomize Mosher's vision for a dignified atmosphere and quiet support for the mentally ill. The assignment of pupils to Pavilion F made their training exceptionally complete. At this point in time, Mosher considered that "nursing was more vital than buildings or drugs."

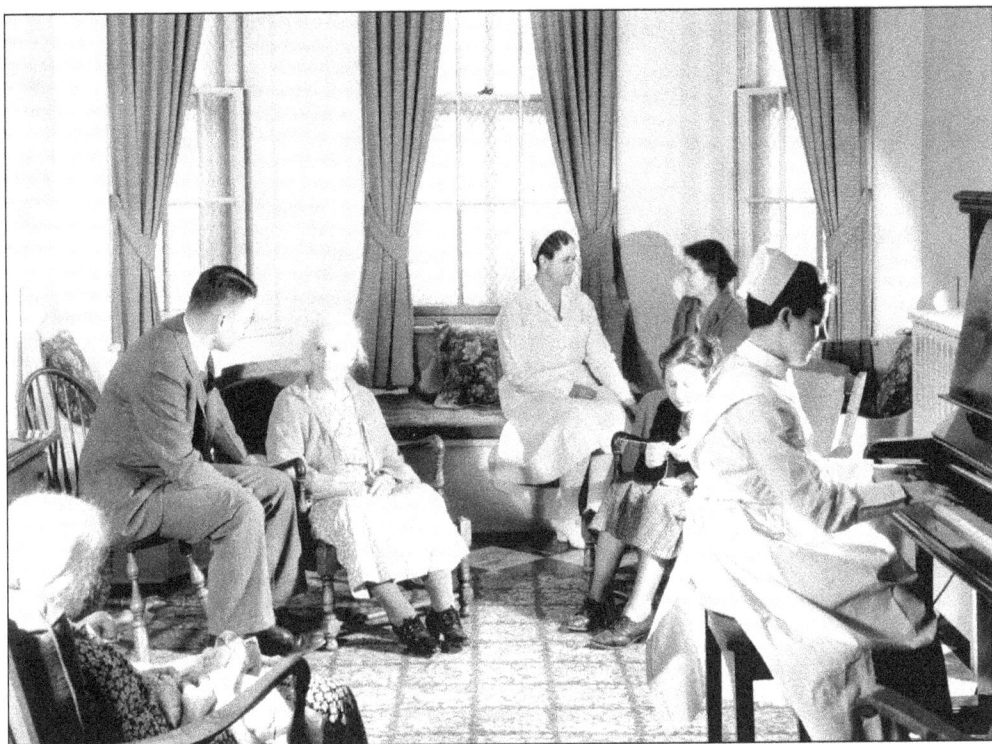

THE DAYROOM ON THE WOMEN'S WARD. Pavilion F was later called Mosher Memorial in honor of the physician whose vision for humane care of the mentally ill is evident in the interaction of patients, doctors, and nurses in the dayroom of the women's ward.

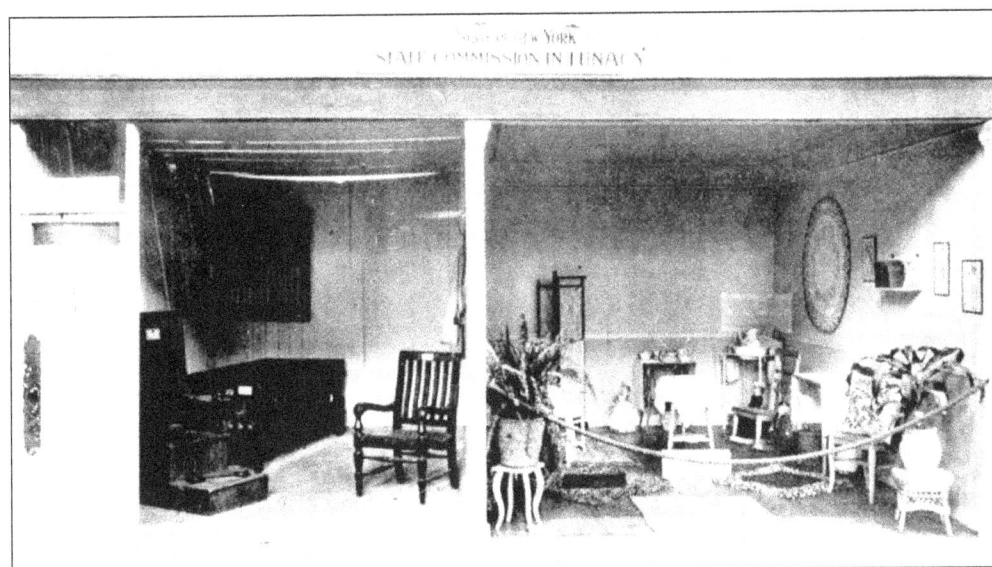

A 1905 ST. LOUIS WORLD'S FAIR EXHIBIT. This exhibit, which contrasted the older stark asylum care of the patient with a restraining chair and the dayroom of the mental ward at Albany Hospital, gained worldwide attention. As a result, similar units were founded in other hospitals. (Courtesy New York State.)

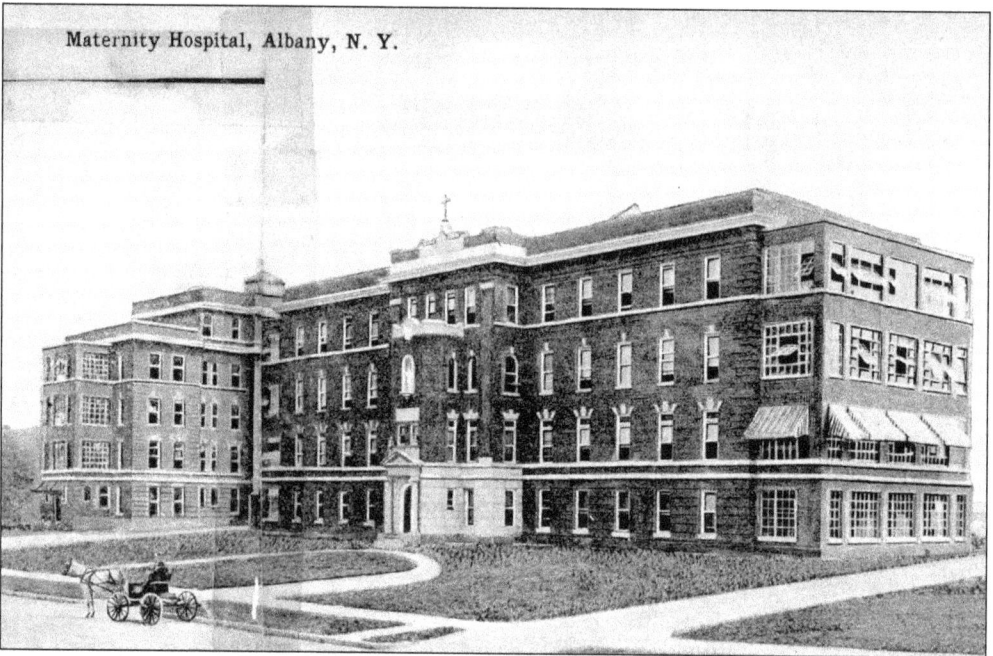

Maternity Hospital, Albany, N. Y.

BRADY MATERNITY. In 1921, Albany Hospital's obstetric census was inadequate. Students averaged only four cases, which was well below the state requirement of 10 cases. This deficit was lessened by an affiliation with Brady Maternity, which provided three months of experience for eight pupils per year. The building still stands on Main Avenue. (Courtesy the Roman Catholic Diocese of Albany.)

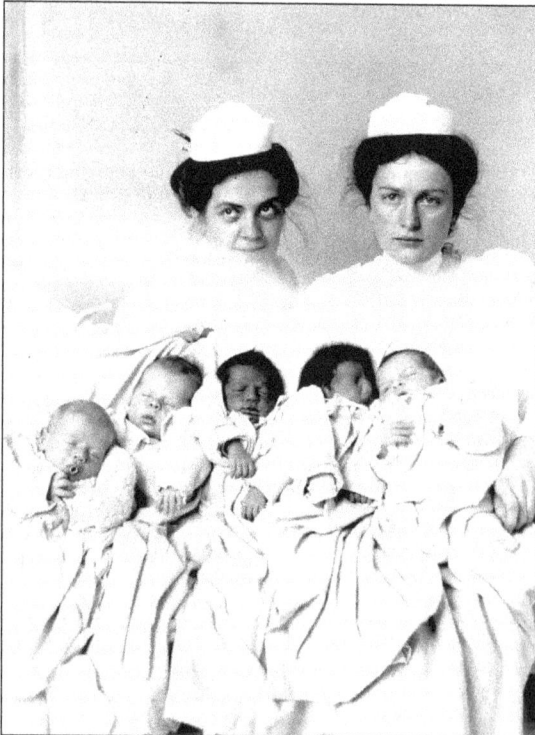

TWO NURSES WITH FIVE BABIES. These nurses needed big laps to hold these peacefully sleeping babies. One has a stuffed-nipple pacifier, and all are abundantly clad in the style of the day.

Newborn Care. This newborn is getting a weight check. Use of a mask was standard procedure for newborn nursery. Cloth diapers were reused through many launderings.

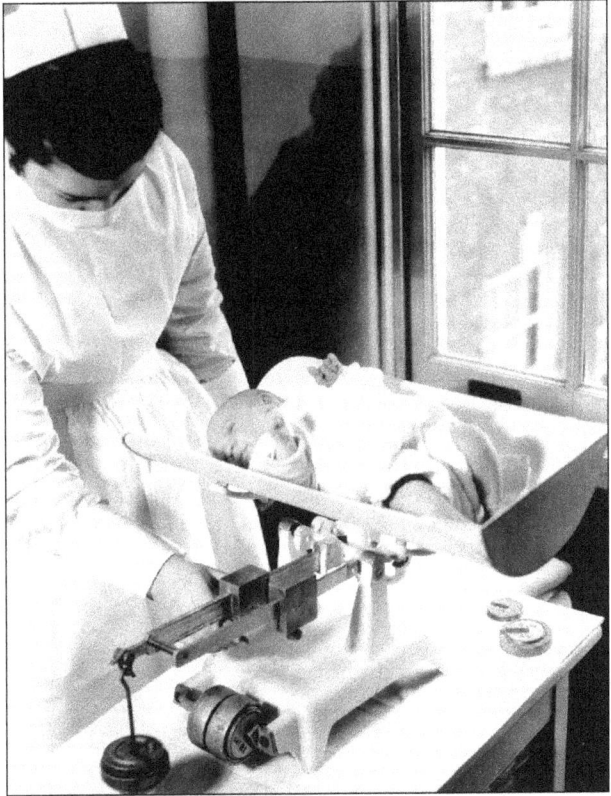

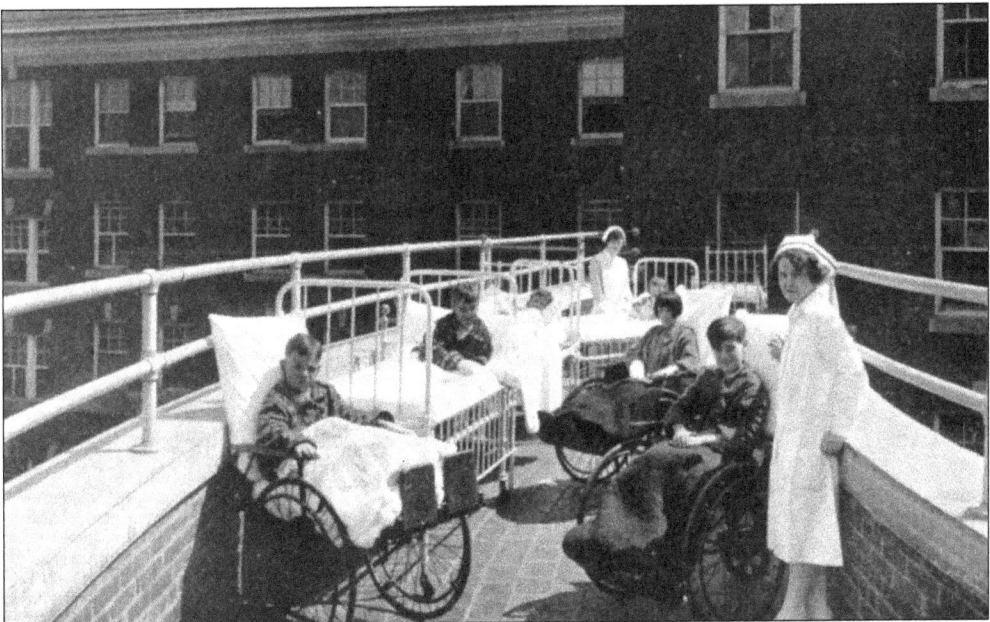

Fresh Air and Sunshine. The outdoor runway was on the roof that connected the nurses' residence with the hospital. It provided a fine area for children who were well enough to be brought outside to benefit from the fresh air and sunshine.

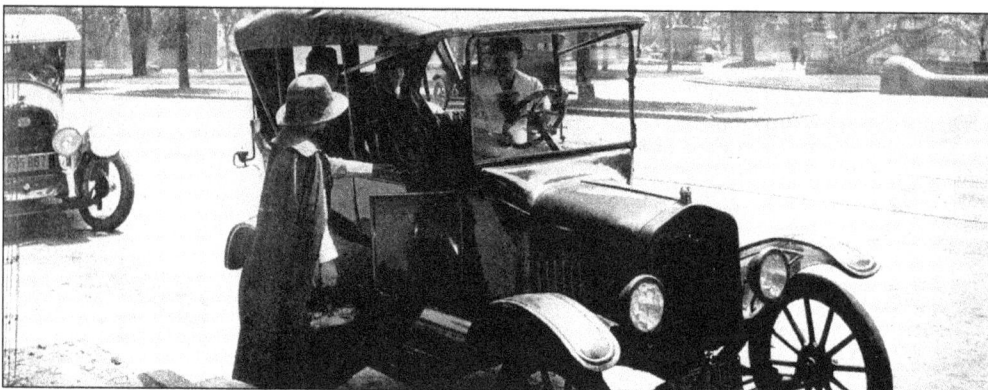

A TAXI FOR PUBLIC HEALTH DUTY. In 1897, the Albany Hospital Limited Means Department was permanently established and student nurses were sent out into the community to provide home care for a period not to exceed three weeks. The next recorded public health activity occurred in 1918, when during the third year of training, a two-month course with the Albany Guild for Public Health Nurses was made an elective.

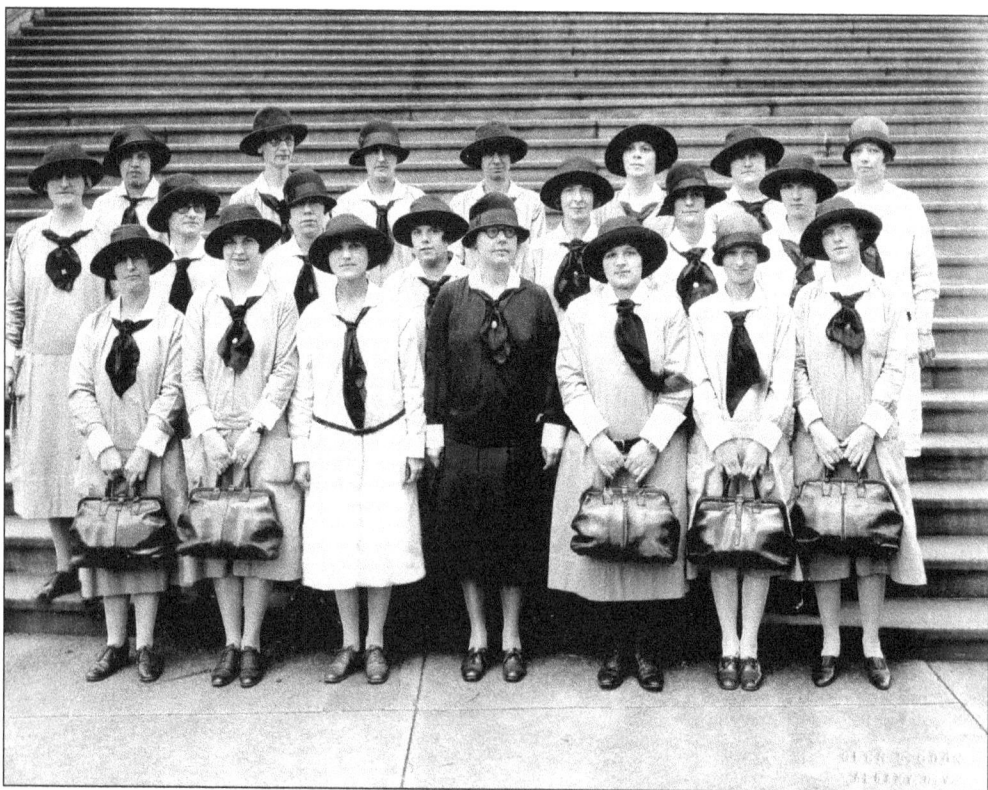

DISTRICT NURSES IN UNIFORM. The dress of district nurses, later known as visiting nurses, might have changed, but the black bag remained their trademark. The district nurses began as a group of philanthropic women known as the Fruit and Flower Guild, which coordinated the delivery of fruit and flowers to shut-ins or to the ill.

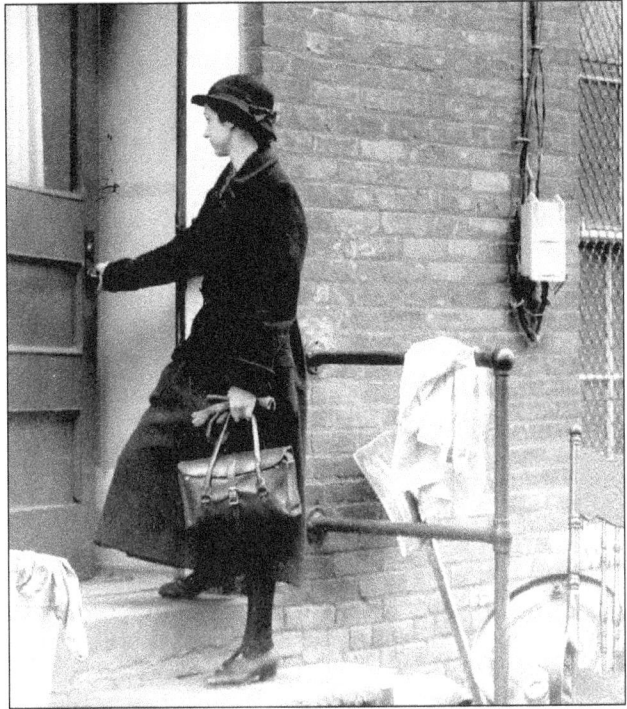

A VISITING NURSE'S ARRIVAL. Recognizing the paramount need of the shut-ins and ill for nursing care, the Fruit and Flower Guild reorganized in 1889 with plans to employ trained nurses. Their aim was educational and preventative, not simply curative. The name has changed too, as the unit was named the Albany Guild for the Care of the Sick Poor, 1896; the Albany Guild for Public Health Nursing, 1919; and the Visiting Nurse Association of Albany (VNA), 1937.

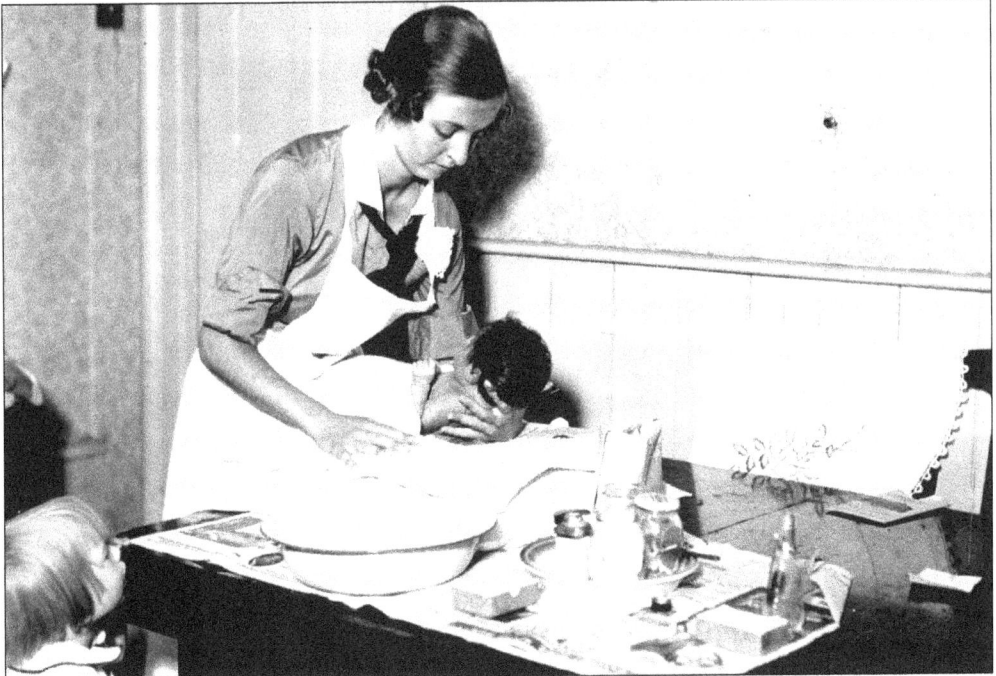

NURSING CARE IN THE HOME. The impact of family members on the patient's care was very evident during a home visit. Note the interest of the toddler. A 1923 report from the New York State Education Department noted that about 75 percent of students received two months of experience in public health nursing, with the remaining 25 percent assigned to the South End Dispensary, an outpatient facility.

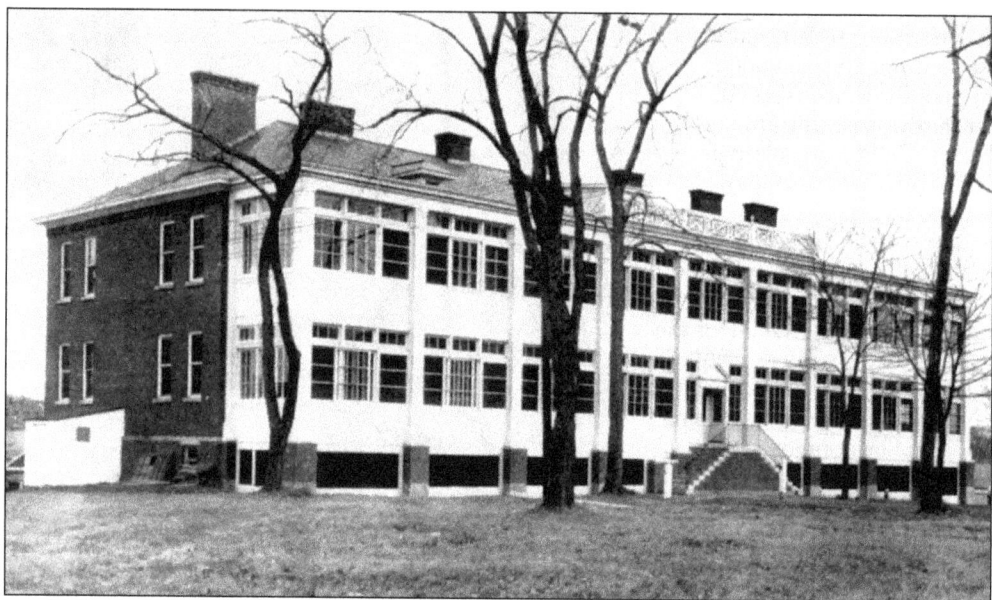

PAVILION G. In 1906, Pavilion G opened, with the school of nursing taking over the nursing care of contagious diseases, including erysipelas, measles, scarlet fever, chicken pox, and diphtheria. The tuberculosis patients who were cared for in tents pitched near Pavilion G were moved to Western Avenue Sanatorium in 1910. Pavilion G was remodeled and named Hun Memorial in memory of Dr. Henry Hun in 1935. Tuberculosis patients received care at Hun Memorial from 1935 to 1974.

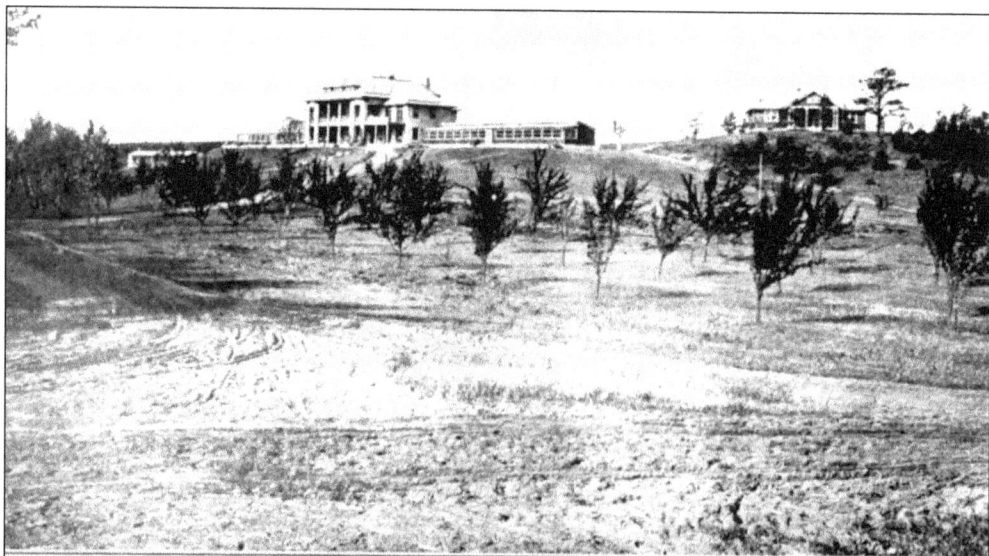

Shacks   The Tuberculosis Sanatorium / Main Hospital   Nurses' Bungalow

WESTERN AVENUE SANITARIUM. In December 1909, the Albany Sanitarium and Red Cross Camp contributed its land, buildings, and equipment to Albany Hospital, which operated and maintained the property for care of tuberculosis patients. The sanitarium building was completed and expanded to include a seven-room bungalow for pupil nurses. A chicken house was installed and work was begun on a piggery.

THE OPEN-AIR WING OF WESTERN AVENUE SANITARIUM. The primary treatment for tuberculosis patients was fresh air and rest. These young patients required extended hospitalization and were taught by teachers from the Albany School District. Although they are in lawn chairs, Adirondack chairs were also used in tuberculosis sanitariums and have maintained their popularity. Records reveal that several pupil nurses contracted tuberculosis.

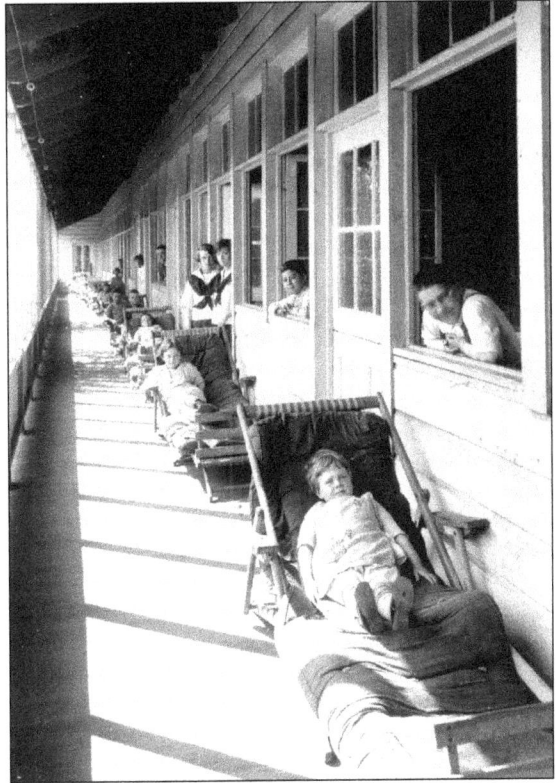

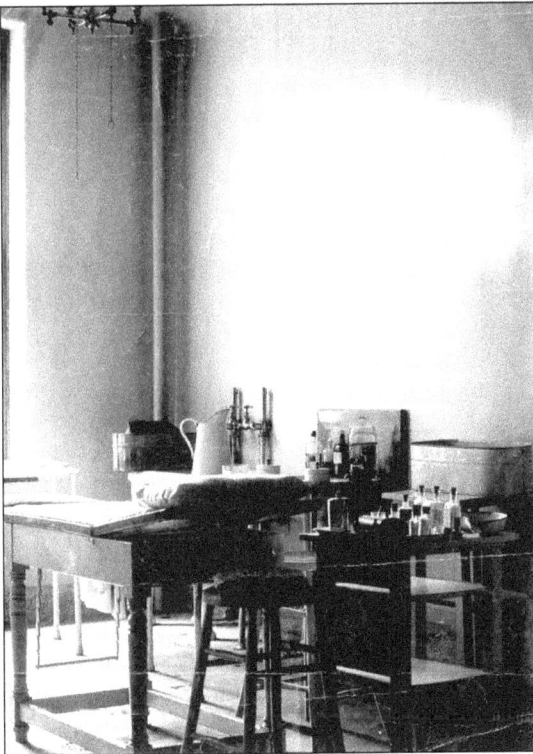

AN OPERATING ROOM FOR SEPTIC CASES, C. 1900. This stark picture recognizes the need to care for septic cases away from the remainder of the hospital.

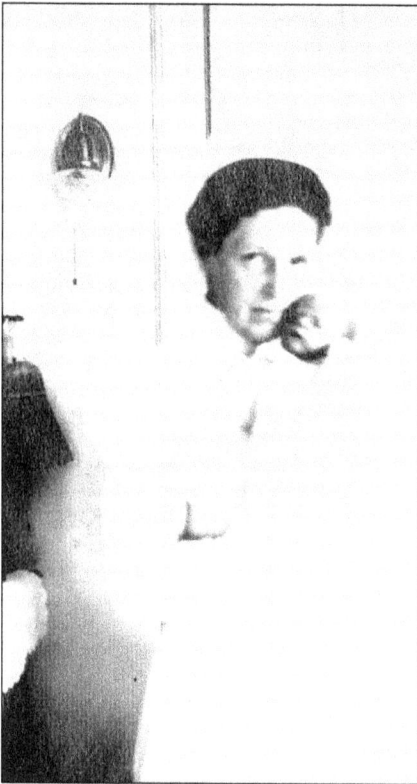

CORNELIA LANSING. Cornelia Lansing, the first probationer, was admitted on January 12, 1897, and signed the agreement on February 13, 1897, to remain for three years (see page 13). She was the first to complete the full three-year course and became the first president of the Alumnae Association. Lansing did private duty, as did many graduates, and specialized in obstetric nursing.

Cornelia Lansing			Jennie Fenton Smith		
Admitted Jan 12 1897			Admitted February 1st 1897		
Graduated May 1900.			Graduated		1900
General ward work	6	15	General ward work	5	36
Operating room		37	Operating room		48
Special nursing		94	Special nursing		49
Night duty	1	36	Night duty	2	65
Sick list		12	Sick list (typhoid)	1	34
Vacation		63	Vacation		63
Obstetrical cases 4			Obstetrical cases 10		
Dietetics Class 6			Dietetics Class 6		
Childs Hospital		36			
Total number of days	10	95	Total number of days	10	95

CORNELIA LANSING'S RECORD OF ATTENDANCE. Each student completed 1,095 days that included 63 days of vacation. Jennie Fenton Smith's total was 1,095. Lansing completed 995, although the total is recorded as 1,095.

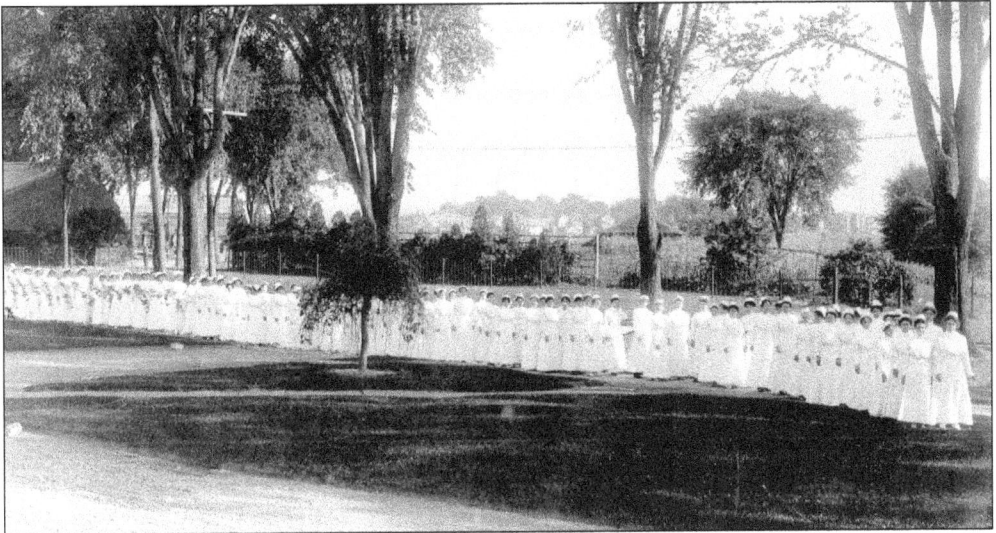

THE 1914 GRADUATION AND REUNION PROCESSION. In 1914, all former graduates were invited to participate in the graduation procession by Susan Hearle, superintendent of nurses, which made it a reunion day as well. The graduates are carrying roses.

...Charges...

Albany Hospital Graduate Nurses

===

1. Private Home cases (4 hours recreation), $30 per week. $4.50 per day less than a week.

2. Hospital Cases, 12 hours duty, $25 per week.

Hospital Cases, 18 hours duty, $4.50 per day.

Hospital cases (12 hour) fraction of a week, $4.00 per day.

3. Mental Cases in private home, $5 per day.

Mental Cases in hospital, $30 per week. $4.50 per day less than a week.

4. Alcoholic Cases (private home) $5 per day.

Alcoholic Cases (hospital) $30 per week. $4.50 per day less than a week.

5. Obstetrical cases, mother and baby, $30 per week; mother or baby, $30 per week.

6. Contagious Diseases, $5 per day. Measles, Scarlet Fever, Diphtheria, Erysipelas, Small-Pox and other Venereal diseases.

7. To prepare patient and room for operation, $5.

8. Laundry to be paid by the patient on cases of contagion and out-of-town cases only.

9. Day of going to the case, day of leaving the case, to be considered separate days excepting where the nurse leaves before 9 a. m.

10. The nurse to be paid from time of engagement, providing she makes it known at the time.

11. When the order for the nurse is canceled after her arrival at the house, she is entitled to one day's pay pro rata.

ALBANY HOSPITAL NURSES' ALUMNAE ASSOCIATION CHARGES. Many graduate nurses did private duty after graduation. Charges for specific types of cases and time spans, c. 1910, were agreed upon through the Alumnae Association.

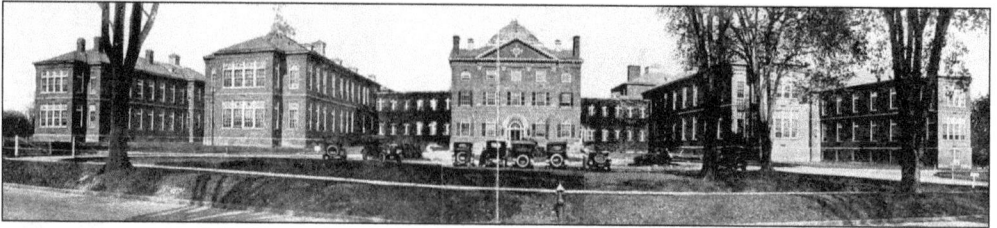

ALBANY HOSPITAL, C. 1914. Albany Hospital accommodated about 185 patients, 100 of whom were to be free patients, and the remainder were private or paying patients. Free and paying departments were separate, as were medical and surgical patients. Eight rooms in Pavilion A had open fireplaces, and two had private baths. The dispensary department was situated in the lower story of Pavilion D for the outdoor relief for the poor.

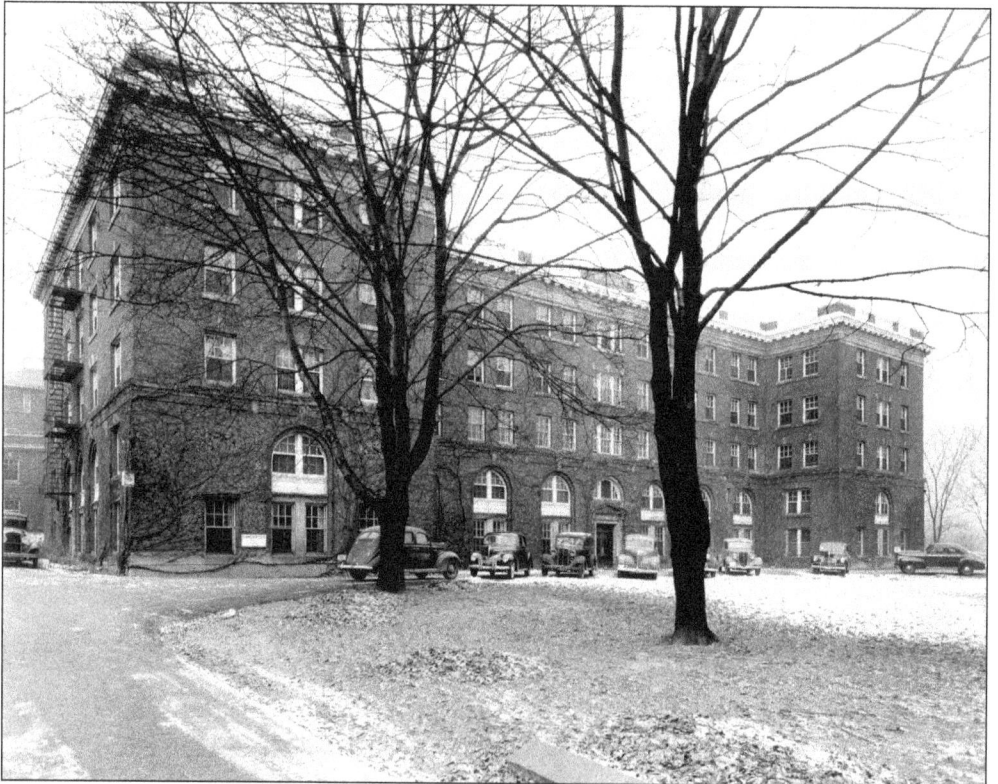

A NEW NURSES' RESIDENCE. Opened in 1914, the residence was a five-story fireproof building connected with the hospital by two enclosed corridors whose gates were locked at night. There were 150 single rooms, 9 marble and tiled bathrooms, 3 marble stairways, a large recreation or lecture hall that doubled as a dining room to accommodate 180 people at small tables, 6 reception rooms, 2 classrooms, a small laundry, and a kitchen. The school had adequate space at last.

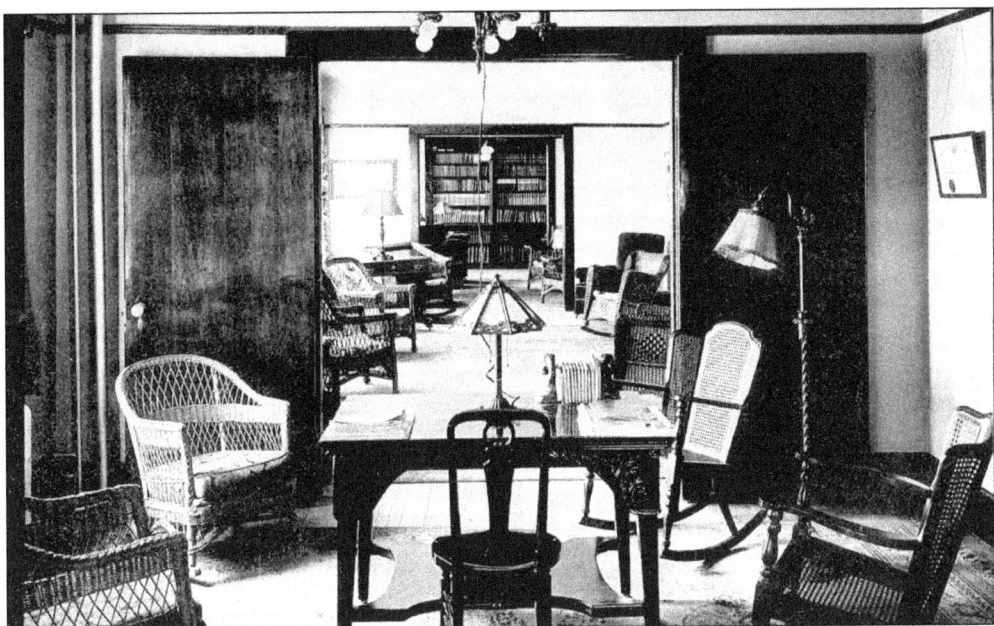

RECEPTION HALLS. Shown are reception halls where guests and friends could be entertained. *The Rules for Nurses* warned, "The Home closes at 10 p.m. All inmates are expected to be within doors at that time. The lights will then be turned off in parlors, halls and bathrooms and each nurse must retire to her own room. All lights in nurses' bedrooms must be turned out at 10:30 p.m."

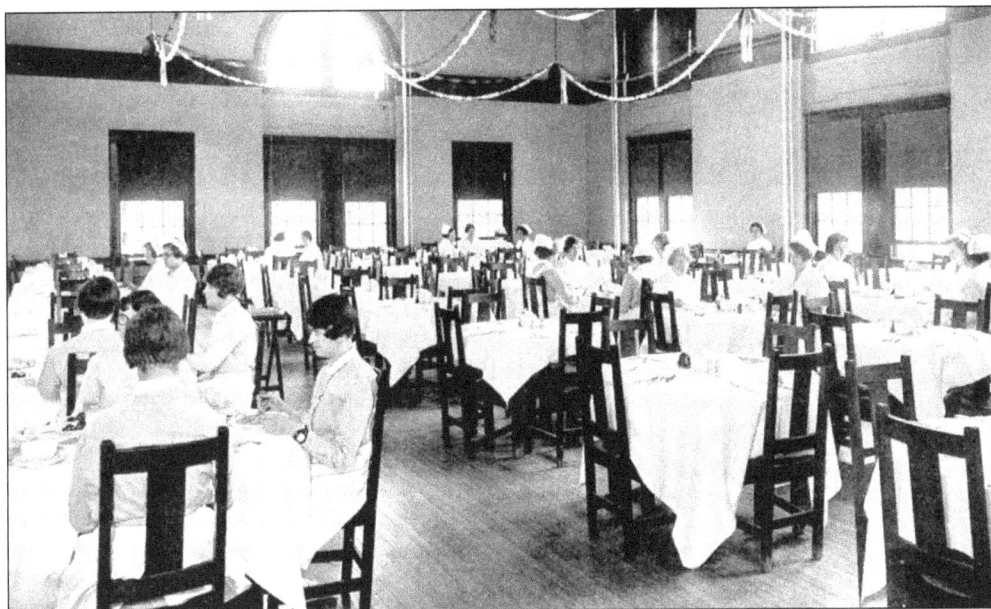

THE RESIDENCE DINING ROOM. In the dining room, a pecking order was evident. No nurse could leave the room if someone her senior were on their feet. Everyone was the probationer's senior. You got up, but rarely did you get to the door before someone your senior was on their feet. When they reached the door, another was up. It was quite an indication of who was liked, resented, or being put in their place.

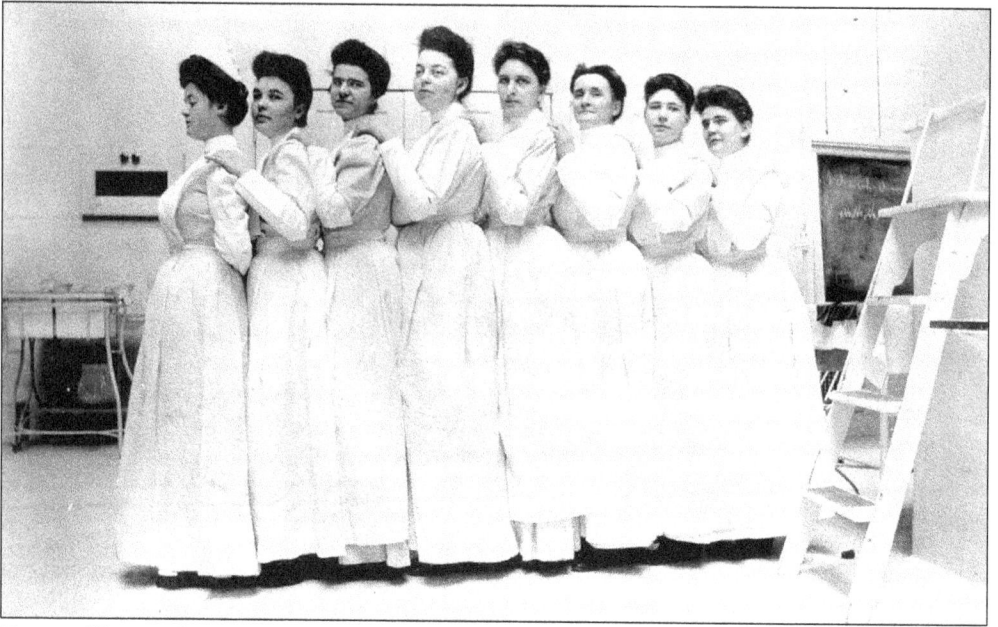

PRETTY NURSES ALL IN A ROW. The first uniform was a pink, ankle-length shirtwaist dress with just-below-the-elbow-length sleeves. The apron, bib, cap, collar, and cuffs were white cotton. Shoes and stockings were black. The cuff, extending from wrist to above the elbow, was pinned to the sleeve, removed during work, and tucked behind the bib. The small stiff collar often caused irritated scratched necks. Later changes included a Peter Pan collar, shorter cuffs, and a shorter hemline.

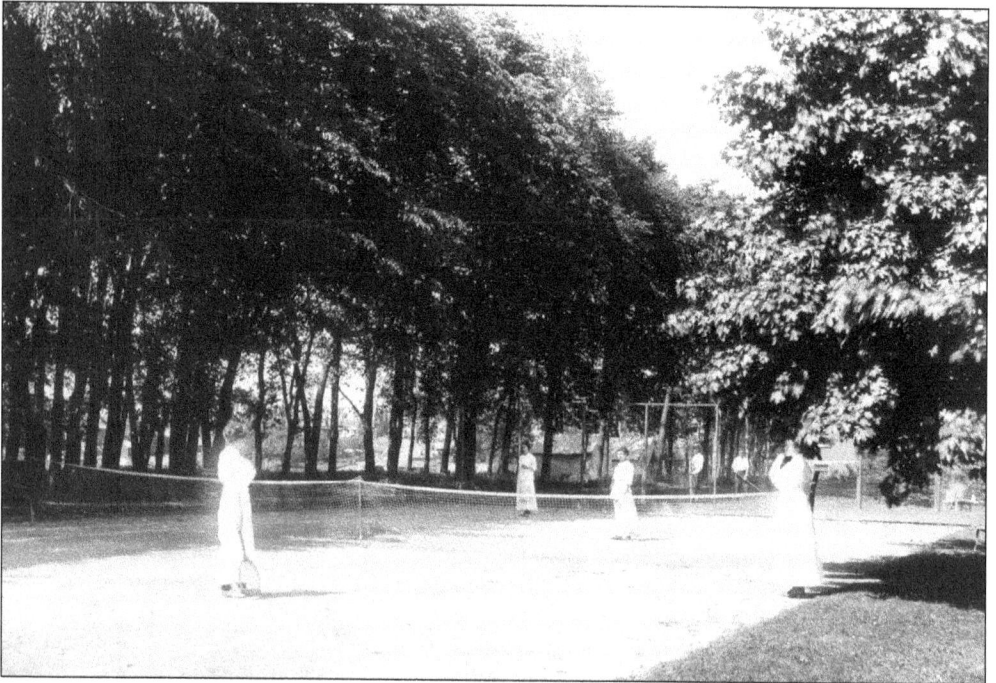

A TENNIS MATCH. Elbow-length sleeves and flat shoes are the only leeway given to these ladies in the garb of the day.

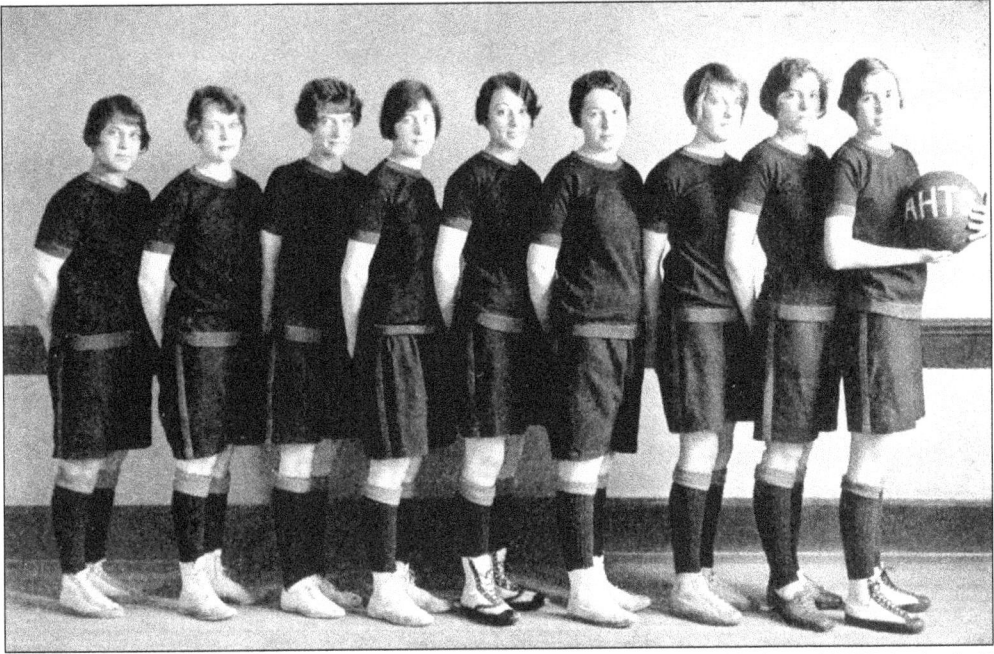

A BASKETBALL TEAM. The 1927–1928 basketball team members hold their AHTS basketball proudly and look quite modern in their uniforms. It would be interesting to know who an opposing team might have been.

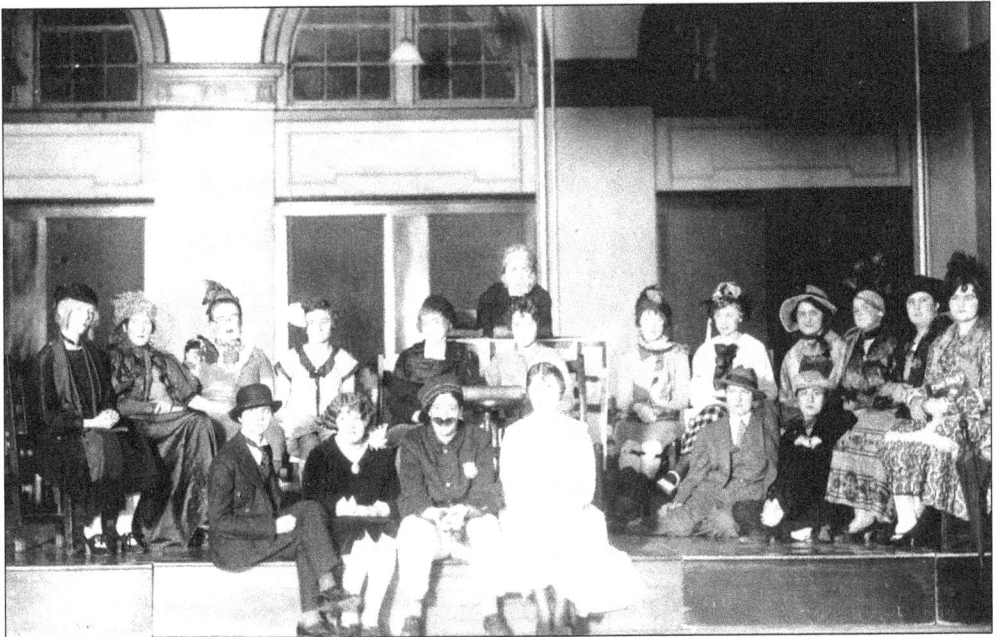

A MINSTREL SHOW. The 1927–1928 minstrel show drew more than 400 to a packed house in the gymnasium of the nurses' residence. A stump speech on women's rights and violin, banjo, and vocal solos were accented by gibes that centered on doctors and other friends in the audience.

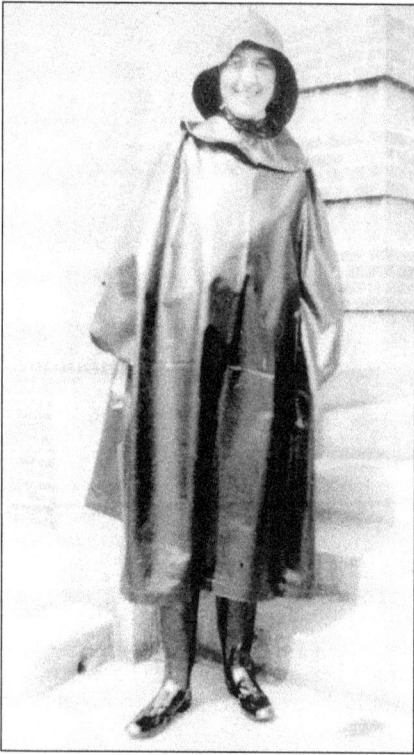

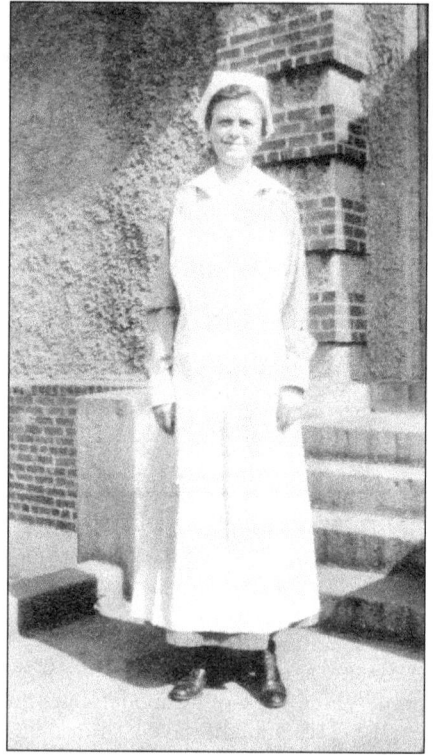

ANNA B. DEGRAFF (1907) AND CORDELIA HILKIE (1909). Anna DeGraff, R.N., wearing her rain slicker, and Cordelia Hilkie, R.N., were among 65 nurses quartered at Ellis Island, living under garrison conditions and receiving intensive instruction in military medicine and surgery as well as instruction from *The Army Hospital's Military Law and Customs*. In England, Anna DeGraff was a strong addition to the hospital staff as superintendent of housekeeping facilities. She also wrote "To Arms! The Call Is Ringing."

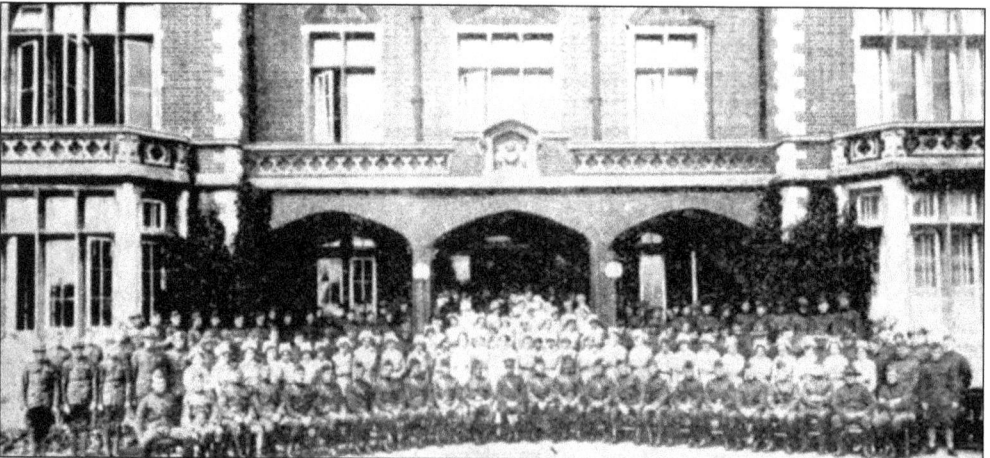

BASE UNIT No. 33 AT PORTSMOUTH, ENGLAND. Personnel for the Albany unit included 24 physicians and surgeons, 152 enlisted men, 65 nurses, and 6 civilians. Equipment included three ambulances, four automobiles, a power-driven wood cutter, a meat chopper, a laundry machine, a fully equipped portable kitchen, two x-ray outfits, and a telephone system. It was planned to have all trades represented in the unit, thus ensuring a truly self-contained group.

36

"To Arms! The Call Is Ringing." This service song of Unit No. 33, U.S. Army Nurses, was written by Anna B. DeGraff (known in some records as Alice A. DeGraff).

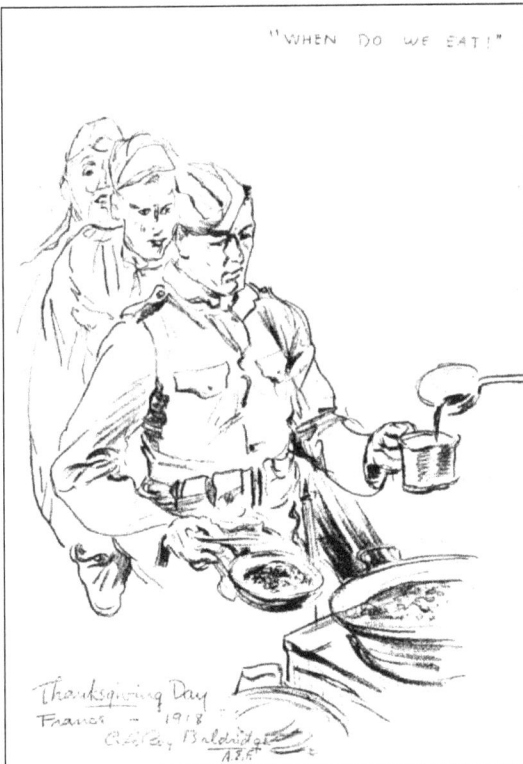

"WHEN DO WE EAT!"

Thanksgiving Day
France — 1918
C.L. Baldridge
A.E.F.

Thanksgiving Day in France, 1918. The artist captures the mood of standing in the mess line at the military base and being away from home even though the armistice had been signed.

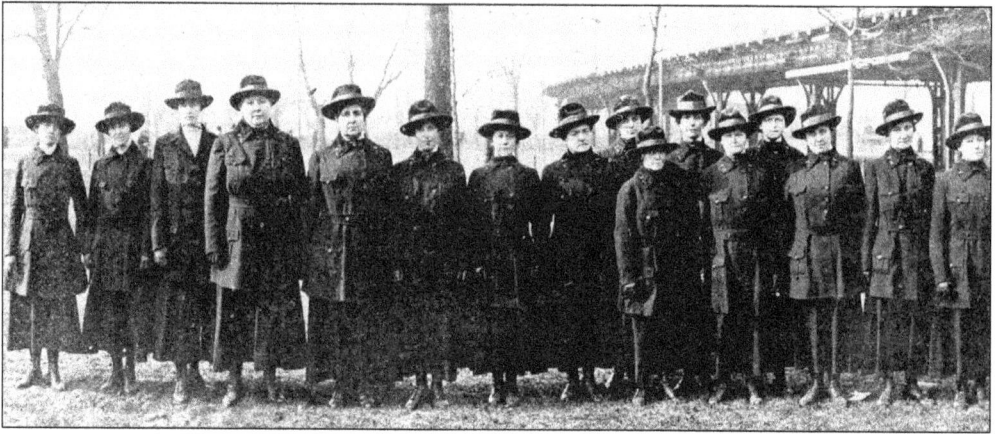

NURSES AND CIVILIANS AT BASE HOSPITAL NO. 33. The board of governors offered the government the services of the hospital, including a base hospital unit for overseas duty, and pledged $33,000 of the total of $114,662 raised from nearby cities, towns, businesses, and Red Cross chapter donations. The first patients admitted, on July 24, 1918, were overseas casualties who arrived by boat at Southhampton, England. On August 2, 1918, Capt. Erastus Corning was placed in command of Base Hospital No. 33 at Portsmouth, England.

Seen above are, from left to right, Irene McKenna, civilian stenographer, Albany; Laura Lipman, civilian stenographer, Albany; Dorothy McCabe, civilian dietitian, Greenwich; Ethyl Walker, Estherville, Iowa; Catherine Kearney, Albany; Evelyn Nisbet, Ithaca; Jean Speirs, New York; Delia Provancher, Mechanicville; Jane Martin (in back), Albany; Sally Ingalls (in back), New York; Cordelia Hilke (in back), Albany; Malvina MacCormack, Albany; Anna Flynn, Albany; Gertrude Roach, Glens Falls; Elsie Kempp, Pittsfield, Massachusetts; and Katherine Lee, Troy.

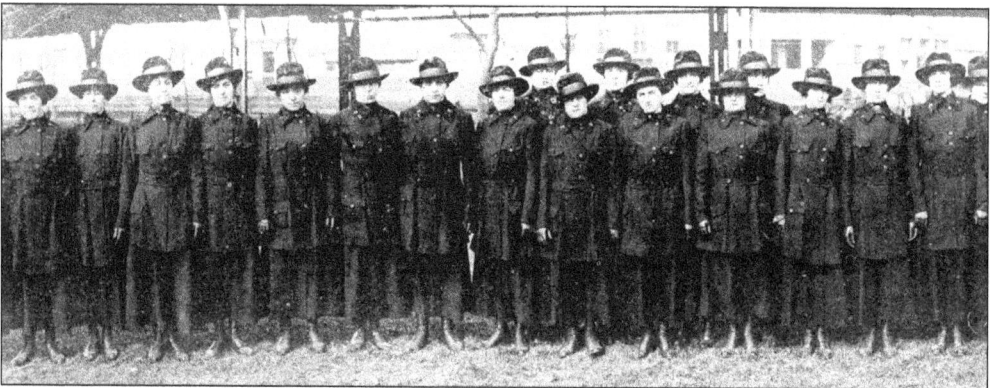

NURSES AND CIVILIANS AT BASE HOSPITAL NO. 33. On the eve of the armistice, Col. Erastus Corning posted a memorandum seeking prayers for "a just and lasting peace." About one-quarter of the total number of graduate nurses still active in nursing served during World War I. About half of this number served overseas.

Shown here are, from left to right, Kathryn Butler, Troy; Florence Heidel, Albany; Helen Clifton, New York; H. Maude Randall, Morton; Florence Burns, Chatham Center; Lulu Guller, Poland; Mattie M. Washburn, chief nurse, Fort Ann; Anna C. Purcell, Herkimer; Gladys Lucas (in back), Gloversville; Florence Tiffany (in back), Rensselaer; Viola Oldford (in back), New York; Mary Kelly (in back), Catskill; Adelaide DeLaMater, Athens; Marion Campbell, Central Bridge; Lillian Yard, Scranton, Pennsylvania; Isabella Brenan, Plattsburgh; H. Marie Riess, Hudson; Bessie Garrah, Albany; and Effie Czerwincki (in back), Buffalo.

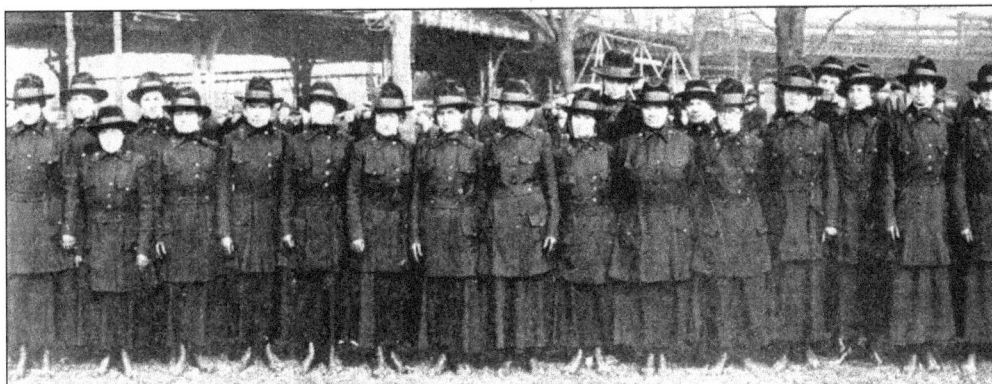

NURSES AND CIVILIANS AT BASE HOSPITAL NO. 33. By the end of September 1918, some 700 patients were being cared for. The influenza epidemic broke out, and within a week, about 800 new cases were admitted to the already crowded hospital. The desperate influenza condition was worsened by an extremely virulent pneumonia. Emergency tents were erected on the countryside with the subsequent transfer of the hospital patients to tents, and the incoming influenza cases centered in the main hospital. Sheets were hung between the beds. While on duty, officers, nurses, and orderlies were ordered to wear long operating gowns, close-fitting caps, and gauze masks, which fitted over their mouths and noses. Nurses were ordered to remain outdoors for two hours daily. Isolation techniques were rigidly observed.

Shown above are, from left to right, Winifred Cosey, North Bennington, Vermont; Anna DeGraff (in back), Albany; D. Amelda Moffett, Schenectady; Lucy Brinkerhoff (in back), Utica, Ohio; Mabel L. Lee, Cohoes; Wilhelmina Hoffman, Schenectady; Stella Hughes, Schenectady; Eleanor Kelly, Schenectady; Eugenia Hinman, Tuscaloosa, Alabama; Flora Graham, Albany; Edith Rushton, Albany; Helen Brooks (in back), Dunkirk; Edith Helen Lowe, Port Ewen; Minnie Tahlman (in back), Albany; Catherine Feeck, Albany; Katherine Quinlan, Pittsfield, Massachusetts; Marguerite Blair (in back), St. Louis, Missouri; Madge Rees, Cohoes; and Christine Gehbauer, Mellenville.

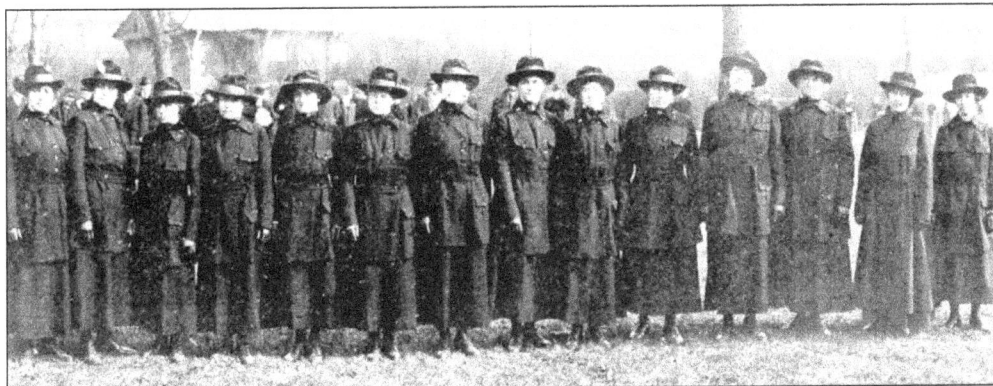

NURSES AND CIVILIANS AT BASE HOSPITAL NO. 33. The Albany unit, with very slight additions to their numbers, gave adequate care continuously to approximately three times the number of patients they were supposed to handle.

Seen here are, from left to right, Anna O'Connor, Albany; Ruth Spencer, Albany; Cora McKay, Albany; Elizabeth Rockstroh, Cooperstown; Edith Chapman, Syracuse; Evelyn C. Dennis, Hudson; Grace DuBois, Schenectady; Mae A. Martin, Watervliet; Dorothy M. Hugo, Amsterdam; Mary McCarty, New York; Marie MacLeod, Hudson; Alice Conlin, Troy; Sara Lane, Schenectady, Lula Lake Harkey, civilian chemist and bacteriologist, New York; and Maud Marshall, civilian stenographer, Albany.

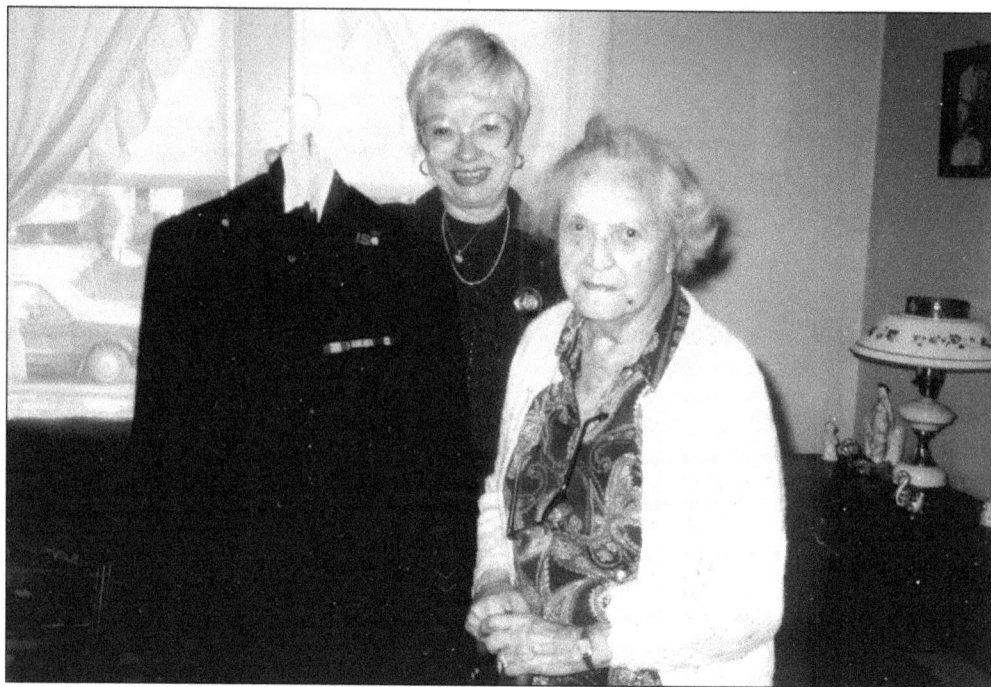

OTILIA NOECKEL BINLEY (1912) DANCED WITH GENERAL PERSHING. Alumni member Sandra Scudder, R.N., Class of 1954, visited with Otilia Binley, R.N., in 1990 and enjoyed her reminiscences of serving in the U.S. Army Nurse Corps in France. Many memories were heart-rending, but one recalling a time of rest and recreation was enthralling. At a dance, wearing the uniform in the photograph, she was held in the arms of one of the most celebrated heroes of World War I, Gen. John Pershing, commander of the American Expeditionary Force (AEF).

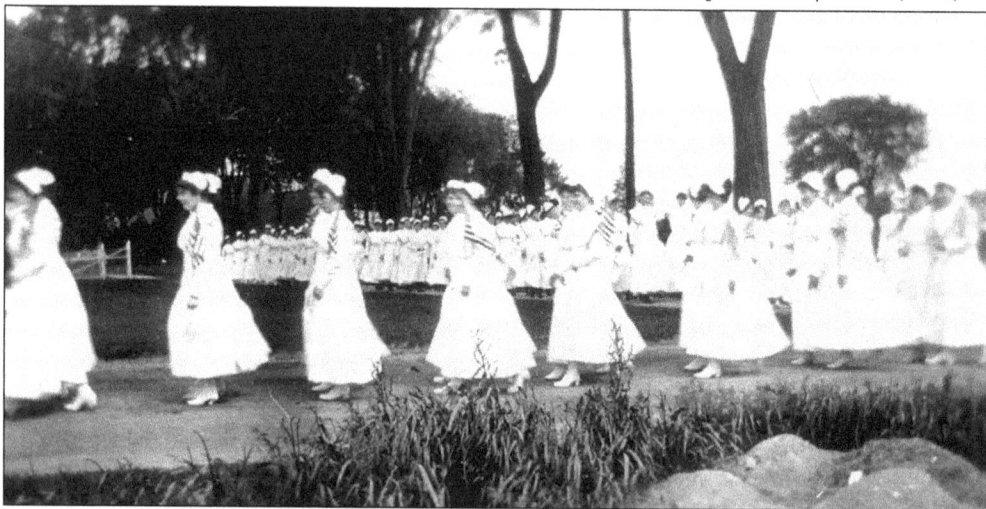

NANCIE CAMERON, CLASS OF 1900. Canadian-born Nancie Cameron, R.N., served at Salisbury Plains training camp in England, at a casualty clearing station in France, and on a ship transporting wounded soldiers home to Canada. She received the Royal Red Cross from King George of England, was given audience with Queen Alexandra, and was cited for "hardships endured and arduous labors in the cause of humanity." In this 1917 photograph, Albany Hospital Training School for Nurses graduates carry their flags proudly.

40

BELL NO. 36 RINGS FOR NURSES. Members of the Nurses' Alumnae Association of Albany Hospital, as well as Memorial and St. Peter's Hospitals, contributed to carillon bell No. 36 at Albany City Hall, "in honor of members who served in the Great War."

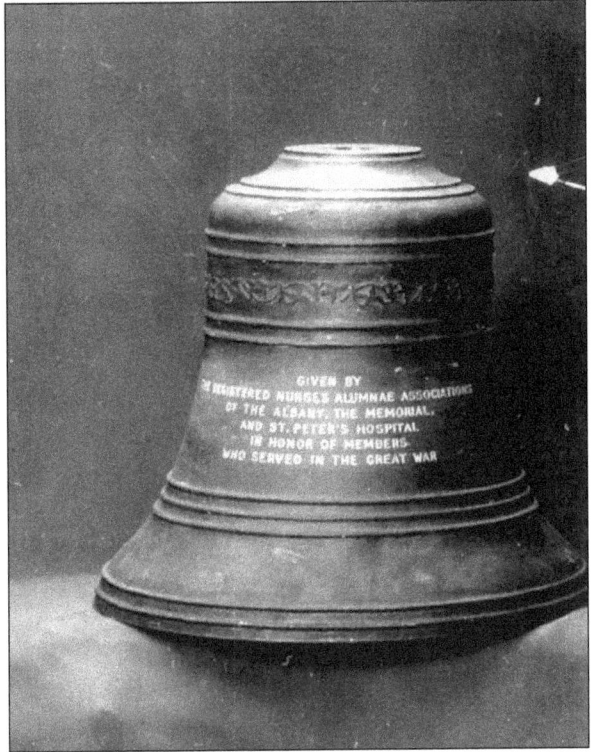

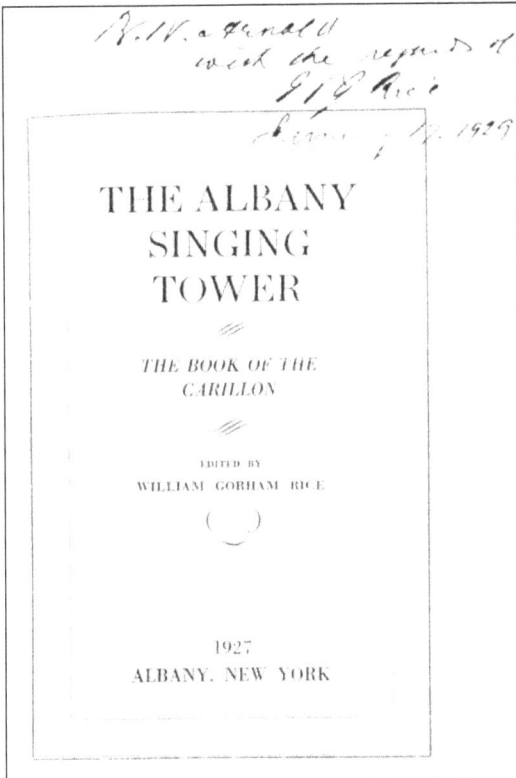

THE ALBANY SINGING TOWER. This was an 80-page memorial booklet with a list of the bells, inscriptions, and names of contributors for the inaugural recital of the 60-bell carillon, given by world-renowned carillonneur Josef Denyn of Belgium on September 18, 1927.

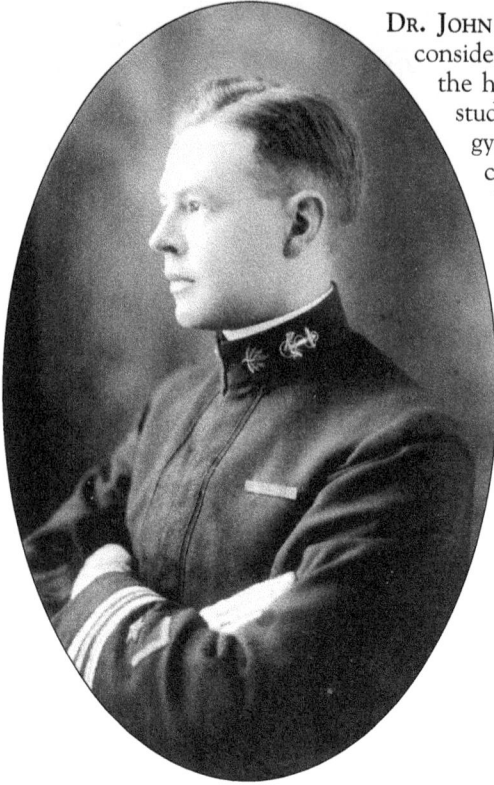

DR. JOHN ALBERTSON SAMPSON. Dr. John Sampson was considered by some to be the patron saint of nurses at the hospital and the AHTSN. His patients and his students loved him. He had worldwide fame as a gynecologist. As a single man, work was his life, colleagues and patients were his family, and the hospital was his home.

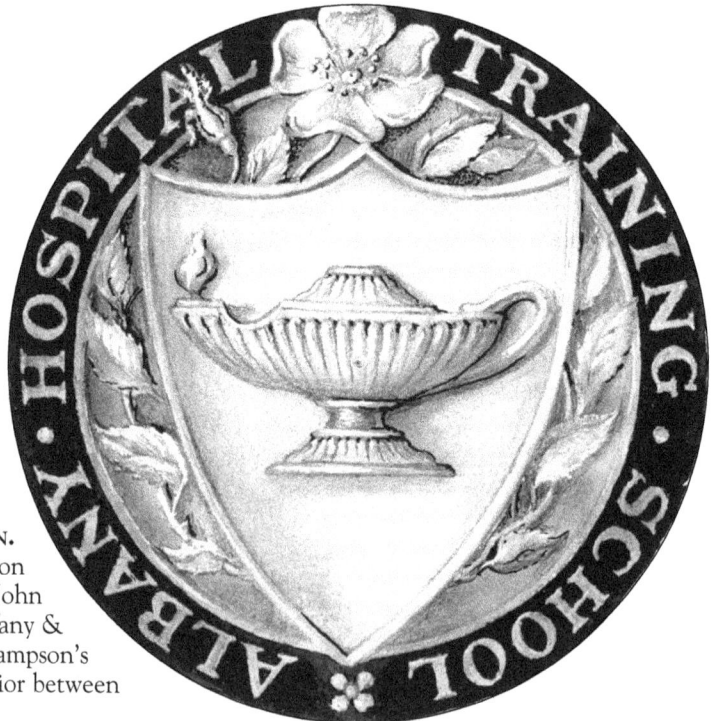

THE GRADUATION PIN. The AHTSN graduation pin was designed by Dr. John Sampson and made by Tiffany & Company. The pin was Sampson's gift to each graduating senior between 1925 and 1937.

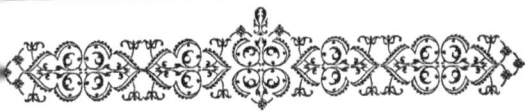

I N designing a pin for you who have received your training in the Albany Hospital Training School for Nurses, it seemed fitting that it should be symbolic not only of the high character of the nursing profession but also of some of the associations and traditions of the Albany Hospital. ⟨ The color of the enamel border in which the name of the training school appears is garnet, chosen from the seal of Union University with which, through the Albany Medical College, your hospital is in close affiliation. ⟨ The rose is the flower of New York State, of which Albany is the capital city. The bud of the rose signifies a promise and the full-blown flower the fulfillment of that promise, as illustrated by the rose you carry at graduation. ⟨ The shield is emblematic of protection, which in your profession is synonymous with prevention

--the prevention of sickness, misery and want. ⟨ The lamp of Florence Nightingale stands for her living spirit which has never failed to light the way to the greatest of all opportunities afforded members of her profession, namely, *service*, the kind of service which only a trained nurse can render, that service which has so greatly contributed, and ever will, to the prevention of disease, the cure of the sick, the healing of wounds, and the comfort of those afflicted.

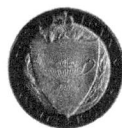

Marion Elizabeth Dunaway

YOU HAVE FULFILLED YOUR PROMISE and with your training you are in a position to help protect yourself and others from needless sickness, misery and want. May the spirit of Florence Nightingale ever be with you and guide you in the great opportunities for service which await you in the practice of your chosen profession.

Mary R. Donald
Supt. of Nurses

THE DIPLOMA OF MARION ELIZABETH DUNAWAY, CLASS OF 1934. Dr. John Sampson's message to the graduates appeared on the diplomas. The diplomas melded the design of the graduation pin with the professional emblems of nursing, using the traditional representations of the state flower in bud and at full bloom and the academic garnet color. Selected symbolism has been carried forward in the pins of Union University School of Nursing and Albany Medical Center School of Nursing. In honor of John Albertson Sampson, the Sampson Award was given to the graduating senior who maintained an outstanding record of excellence in bedside nursing. Marion Dunaway, R.N., was a lieutenant in the U.S. Army Medical Corps with the 33rd General Hospital. Albany Hospital was always her place of civilian nursing employment.

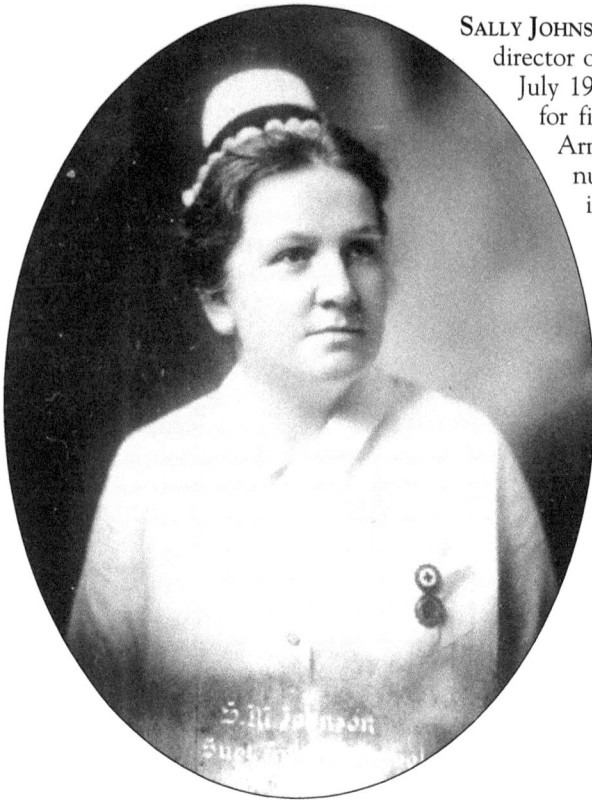

SALLY JOHNSON, R.N. Johnson served as the fourth director of the AHTSN from 1917 to 1920. In July 1918, she was released from the school for five months and assigned by the U.S. Army Nurse Corps as director of the nursing school at Walter Reed Hospital in Washington, D.C. She authored *Historical Sketches*, the training school's history from 1891 to 1920. Hearsay credits her with the design of the organdy AHTSN graduation cap.

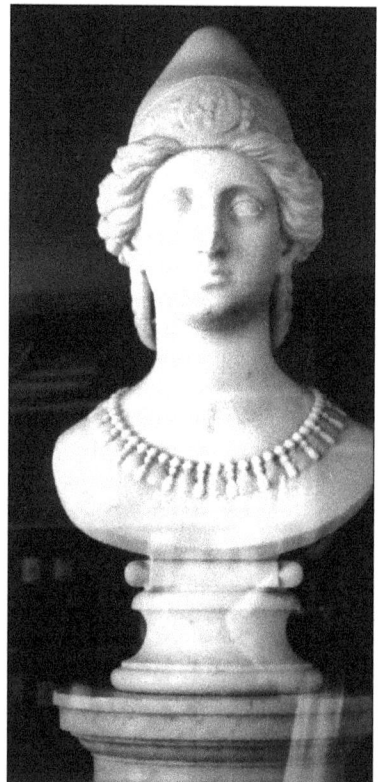

CYBELE. Oral history relates that this statue was known to represent Cybele, the mother-goddess of fertility. It was thought improper to have such a goddess in the nurses' residence, and she was known instead as Minerva, goddess of wisdom. Minerva could be found mysteriously adorned with earrings or tucked into one of the infirmary beds. She is now in the Main 4 solarium as part of a nursing history display.

KATHRYN MACKAY LAMB, R.N., CLASS OF 1914.
Kathryn Lamb was Alumnae Association president during the strike that occurred after a group-nursing policy was instituted without consulting the Nurses' Alumnae Association. The policy allowed two patients to share the same private-duty nurse. Registered nurses walked out of the hospital. Practical nurses and Canadian nurses were hired to maintain nursing service. Many nursing students transferred to other schools. A petition to revoke the licenses of eight nurses was filed.

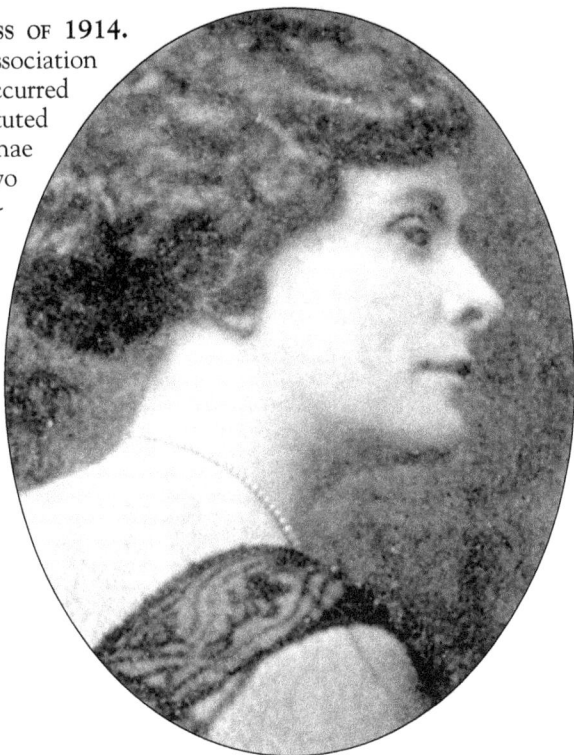

The University Of The State Of New York.

The State Department of Education.

Albany.

Augustus S. Downing
    Assistant Commissioner
    And Director of Professional Education.

March 11, 1926.

John J. McManus, Esq.
Attorney at Law
51 State St.
Albany, N.Y.

Dear Mr. McManus:

I have pleasure in advising you that at a meeting of the Board of Regents held February 19, 1926 the following vote was taken:

"Voted, That the charges preferred against the following named licensed nurses, Kathryn Quinlan, Laura Conway, Margaret MacLucas, Katryn Cosgrove, Edith Lowe, Anna Goldsmith, Mrs. E.A. Lamb, and Mrs. William Bright, and the petition for the revocation of their licenses and of the registration of such licenses, be and the same are hereby dismissed"

                    Very sincerely yours,

                    Agustus S. Downing R.

Note:

    Each of the above named, all the officers of the Alumnae Association, received a copy of this final report.

Kathryn M (Gilbert) Lamb
President of Albany Hos.
Nurses Alumnae Asso.

THE BOARD OF REGENTS DROPS THE CHARGES. After legal proceedings on both sides, a letter was received by the Alumnae Association's attorney that the state board of regents had dismissed the charges against the eight nurses. The copied letter, seen here, has a note stating that Kathryn Lamb sent each officer of the Alumnae Association named in the petition "a copy of this final report."

45

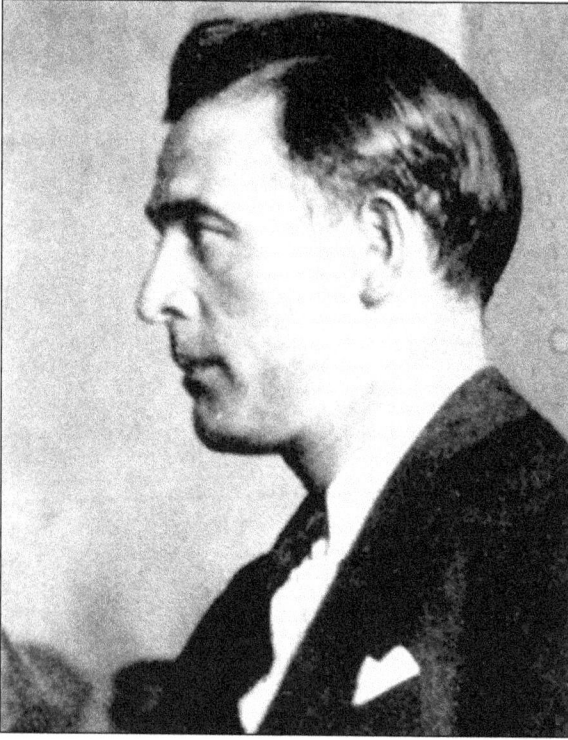

JACK "LEGS" DIAMOND. The notorious gangster Legs Diamond was a patient in the hospital when Daisey Hommel Place, Class of 1933, was a student. He was guarded by state troopers who frequently shared sandwiches they brought in with the staff. Place remembers being caught in the act of eating one of the sandwiches and receiving a reprimand from the supervisor, Hattie McQueen. (Courtesy William Kennedy.)

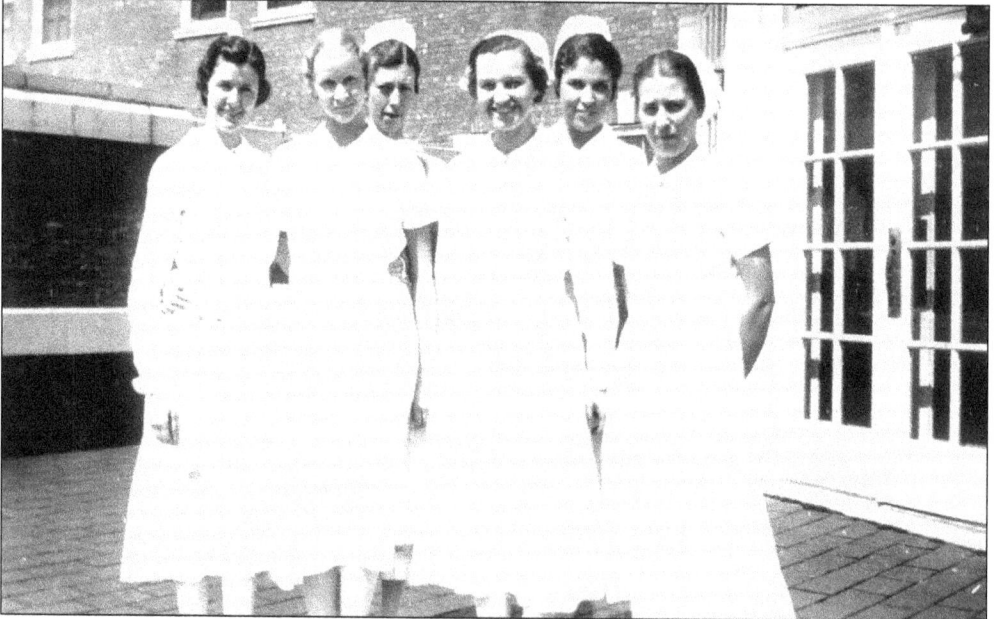

DAISEY PLACE, R.N., CLASS OF 1933, AND CLASSMATES. Pictured here are, from left to right, ? Prosner, R.N.; M. Catherine Baker, R.N.; Daisey Hommel Place; "Buz" Balinski, R.N.; Margaret Lindsay, R.N.; and an unidentified person. The stock market had crashed, but spirits soared among these graduates of the Class of 1933 as they learned, worked, and played in the heart of New York. Seventy years later, class members have remained in touch, still attending alumni reunions. (Courtesy Daisey Place.)

Forever Picking up Toys. This cartoon from the book *Nurse Please! Highlights in the Training of Susie*, by Jean McConnell, depicts one of the timeless challenges that the nursing student faced and attempted to surmount. (Courtesy Lippincott, Williams & Wilkins.)

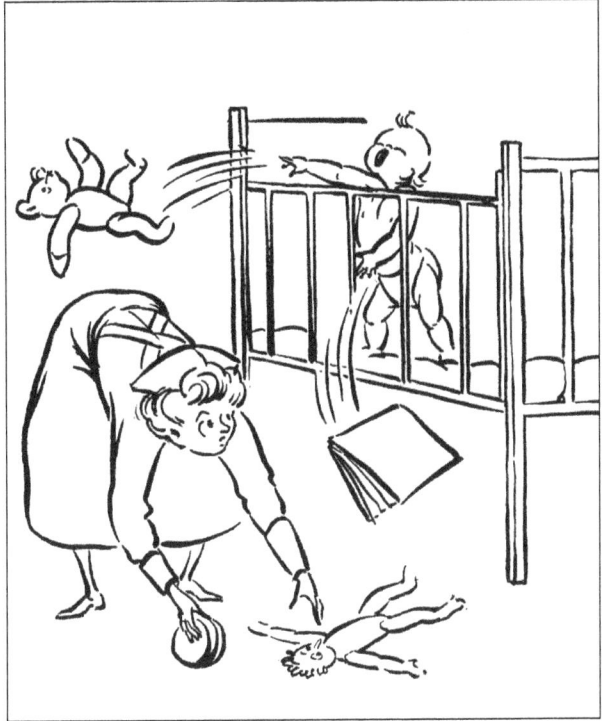

-:- *Care Of Sick*

MISS OLIVINA SPRINGER
THE RIGHT TWIST — One must get in making a hot pack for the patient is demonstrated by Miss Olivina Springer, who will instruct a class of Girl Scouts.

Home-Care Classes. The water is so hot it must be wrung out with handles attached on either side of the hot pack. Olivina Springer, R.N., Class of 1923, will teach the Girl Scouts safety measures for this procedure. (Courtesy *Times Union*.)

NURSING

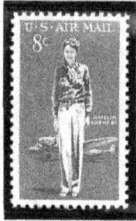

AMELIA EARHART ISSUE
Date of Issue: July 24, 1963
Amelia Earhart was a World War I Voluntary Aid Detachment nurse in Toronto until she became ill during the influenza epidemic. She was the first woman aviator to cross the Atlantic.

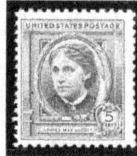

LOUISA MAY ALCOTT ISSUE
Date of Issue: February 5, 1940
Famous as the author of Little Women and other popular novels of her day, Louisa May Alcott also published Hospital Sketches, based on her letters written when she was a Civil War nurse in charge of a ward.

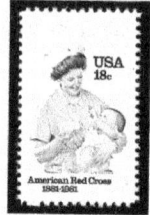

AMERICAN RED CROSS CENTENNIAL
Date of Issue: May 1, 1981
The latest stamp to honor the Red Cross nurses was issued for the celebration of the American Red Cross Centennial.

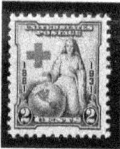

RED CROSS ISSUE
Date of Issue: May 21, 1931
Issued on the 50th anniversary of the American Red Cross, this was the earliest U.S. stamp depicting a nurse. Reproduced from a 1930 poster entitled "The Greatest Mother."

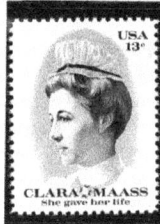

CLARA MAASS ISSUE
Date of Issue: August 18, 1976
Clara Maass served as a nurse with the US Army during the Spanish-American War. Because she felt she would be more valuable as a nurse if she developed an immunity to yellow fever, she volunteered to be bitten by a mosquito thought to carry the disease. She survived but volunteered to be bitten again. She died 10 days later at the age of 25, the only nurse to die during the experiments which led to the conquest of the disease.

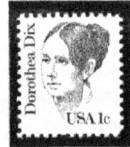

DOROTHEA DIX ISSUE
Date of Issue: September 23, 1983
Appointed as Superintendent of the Female Nurses of the Union Army during the Civil War, Dorothea Dix organized hospitals, assigned nurses, and directed medical supply distribution to the wounded troops. Although she had no formal nursing training, she revolutionized care of the mentally ill, and was honored for her humanitarian efforts.

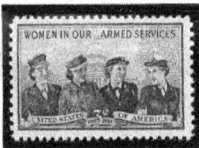

SERVICE WOMEN ISSUE
Date of Issue: September 11, 1952
The United States issued this stamp, the third featuring nurses, to honor women in the armed forces.

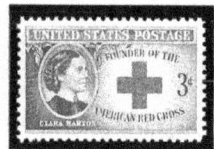

CLARA BARTON ISSUE
Date of Issue: September 7, 1948
A founder of the American Red Cross in 1881, Clara Barton (1821-1912) served as a nurse in the Civil War and the Franco-Prussian War. She directed relief work during floods, famine, fever epidemics, and, at age 76, the Spanish-American War.

THE STAMPS OF NURSING. These stamps name nurses who have attained renown for their outstanding achievements and dedication to the causes they upheld. Louisa May Alcott was also the noted author of *Little Women*. Amelia Earhart gained fame as an aviatrix. In 1932, she was the first woman to fly solo and, at that time, achieve the fastest flight across the Atlantic Ocean.

Two

The Evolution of Nursing Education and Practice

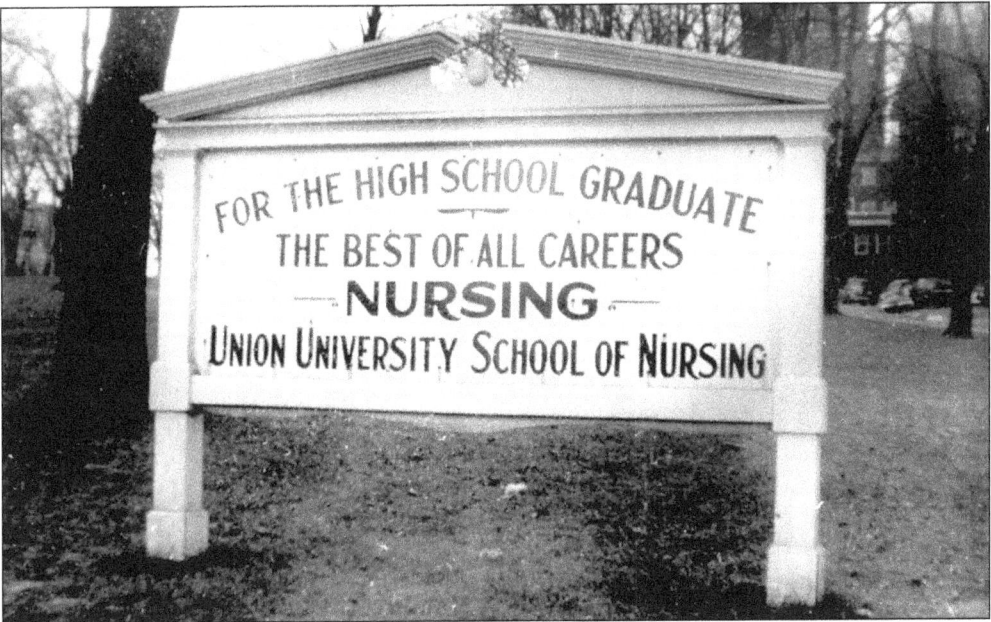

Nursing Education Expands to the College Campus. In the period between 1934 and 1989, hospital nursing evolved from private-duty nursing to the functional method of task-oriented nursing assignments to team nursing. Accordingly, nursing moved from a technical vocation to a profession with the professional nurse educated in the arts and sciences of nursing as well as maintaining proficiency in nursing techniques. In 1982, nursing was acknowledged as an autonomous profession with the passage of the Nurse Practice Act, which distinguished between nursing practice and medical practice. Fewer nurses were entering practice from hospital nursing schools while more were graduating from associate or bachelor of science degree programs. Similar changes were evident in the various nursing programs at Albany Hospital. Russell Sage College School of Nursing (RSCSN) was a collegiate program from 1934 to 1945. The U.S. Cadet Nurse Corps (1942 to 1947), in affiliation with RSCSN, the hospital, and Albany Medical College, was a diploma or collegiate program, as was Union University School of Nursing (UUSN) from 1945 to 1957. AMCSN, which operated from 1955 to 1989, was a diploma program under the board of governors at Albany Hospital. (Courtesy Eina Conde O'Dea, R.N., Class of 1955.)

SCHOOL SONG

Alma Mater - Union University School of Nursing

1. FROM FARMS AND CI-TIES FAR AND NEAR, WE LEFT OUR HOMES TO US SO DEAR,
2. OUR FOND-EST THOUGHTS WILL EV-ER BE, WITH UN-ION UN-I-VER-SI-TY,

WE KNOW THE GOALS WE SET ARE HIGH, THEY WILL BE REACHED IF WE BUT TRY
OUR STU-DENT DAYS OF WORK AND PLAY, WILL EV-ER IN OUR MEMORIES STAY

TRA-DI-TIONS OLD WE WILL UP-HOLD, AS DOWN LIFES PATH WE WEND OUR WAY
OUR HEARTS ARE TRUE IN ALL WE DO, AS DOWN LIFES PATH WE WEND OUR WAY

THE UNION UNIVERSITY SCHOOL OF NURSING ALMA MATER. Throughout the years, young women did indeed come to Albany Hospital from "farms and cities far and near" to reach the goal of becoming registered nurses. UUSN became a division of Albany Medical College in 1945. UUSN students were offered the opportunity to earn a nursing diploma or, with 60 additional credits from any liberal arts college, were awarded a baccalaureate degree in nursing from Union University.

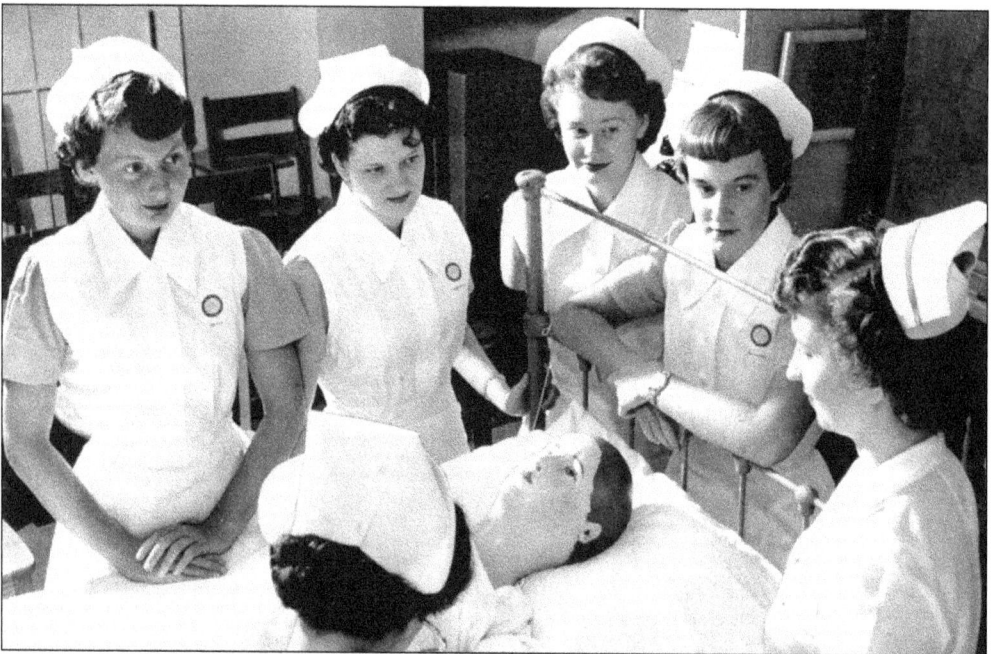

MRS. CHASE. What new procedure will Mrs. Chase have practiced on her today? Practice was done in the classroom. After the task was satisfactorily completed in the clinical area three times under instructor supervision, the student was allowed to perform the procedure on a patient without supervision.

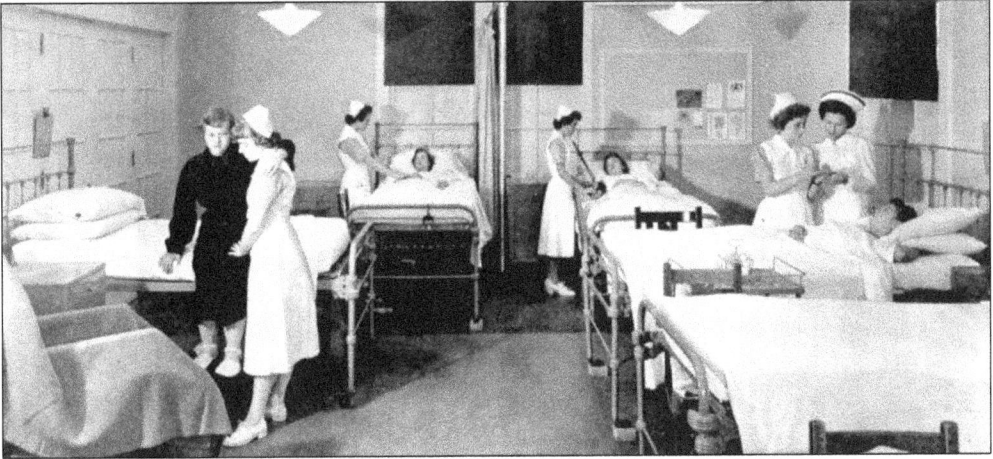

A CLASSMATE BECOMES MRS. CHASE. In the nursing arts classroom, practice began as students assumed the role of patient or nurse. Within three weeks after entering the school, students were ready to go on to the wards for patient care. They started with becoming acquainted with the ward, visiting patients, and fixing flowers. After each classroom practice, more patient care was added.

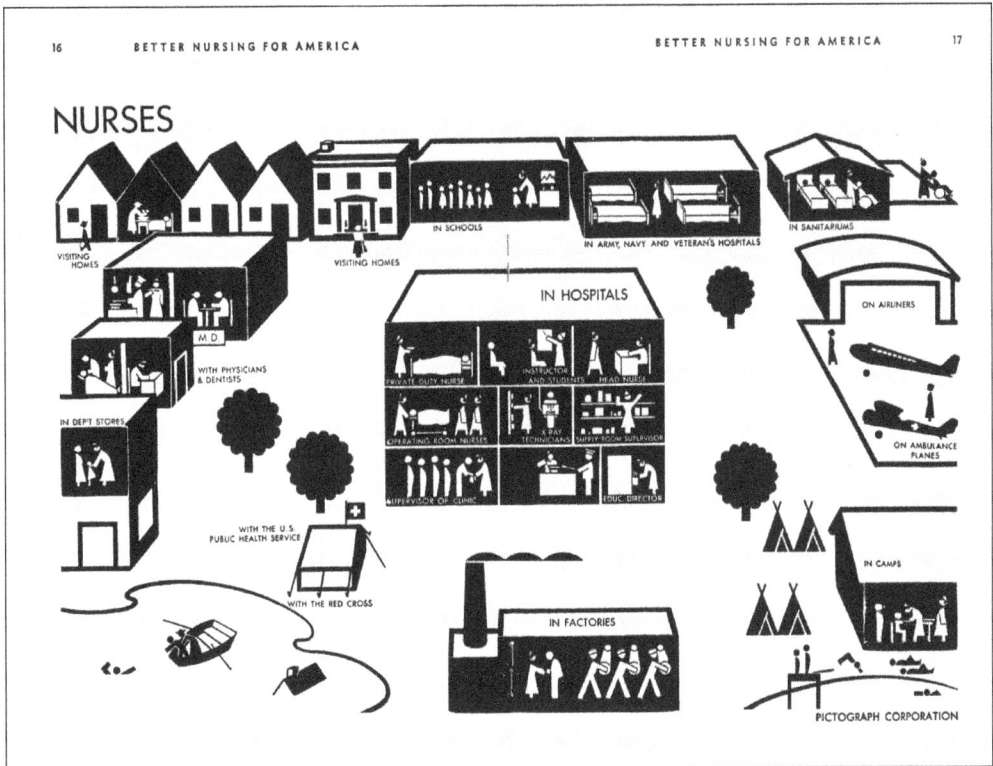

THE MANY FACES OF NURSING. While hospitals provided many opportunities for nursing skills, nursing services also expanded into the community, as shown in this 1941 pictogram in the public affairs pamphlet *Better Nursing for America*, by Beulah Amadon.

51

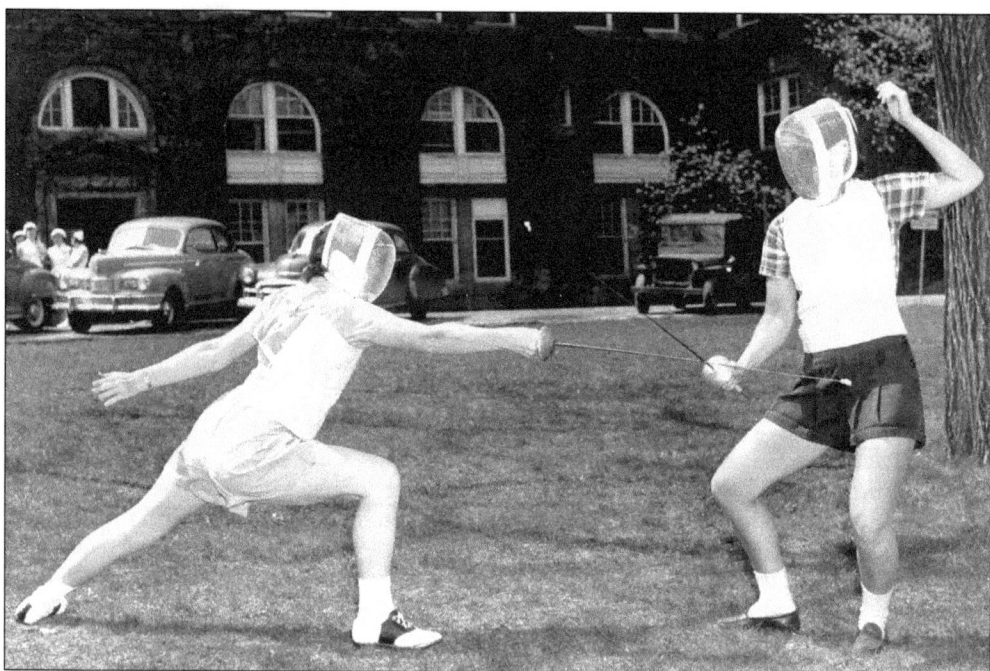

ON GUARD. These nurses are fencing on the nurses' residence lawn during their time of rest and relaxation. Other recreation choices included sports engagements, theater, a library, music, and museums, which have always been abundant in the Albany area.

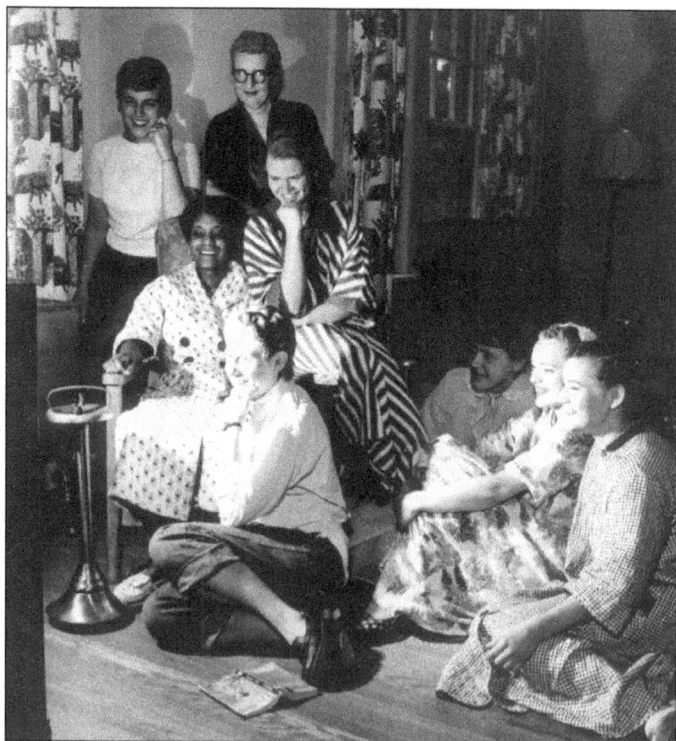

TELEVISION, C. 1956. With the advent of television, hours were spent in the living room sitting around the set with classmates and friends. Housemother Lois Stewart also enjoyed watching.

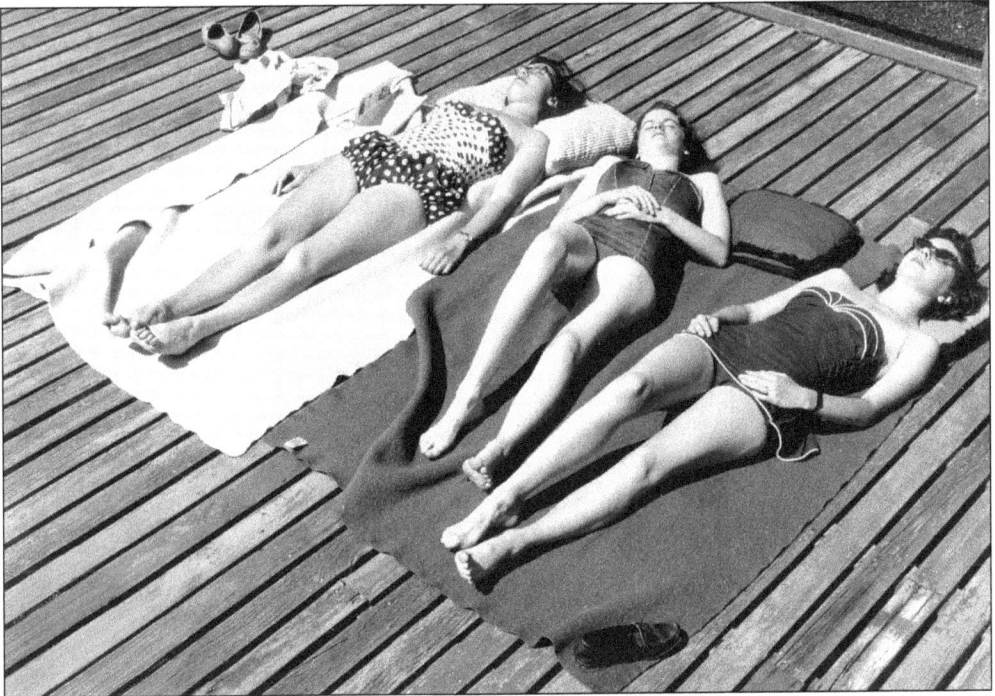

SUNBATHING. The housemother was just as overjoyed as the students when she put in a requisition for a sundeck on the roof of Bolton Hall, and it was approved and built. Students from other residences could sunbathe there as well. It was also a popular spectator sport from vantage windows in the hospital.

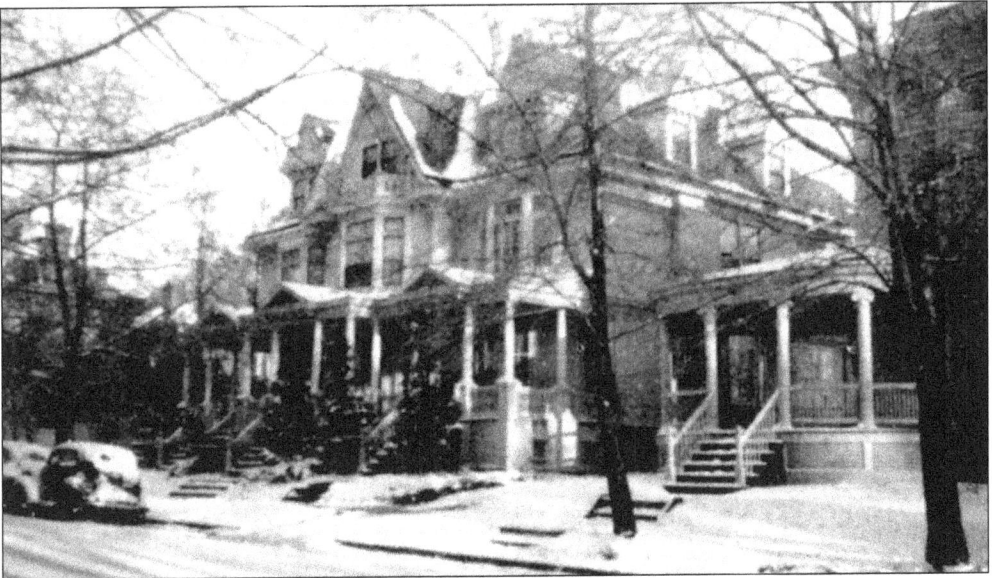

WREN HALL. In September 1949, 27 women and 15 men from Harlem Valley, Binghamton, Middletown, and Marcy State Hospitals, which were under the direction of the New York State Department of Mental Hygiene, began a one-year affiliation at Albany Hospital and UUSN for medical and surgical, operating room, obstetric, and pediatric nursing. Wren Hall, located on 100–104 South Lake Avenue, was the residence for these first male students.

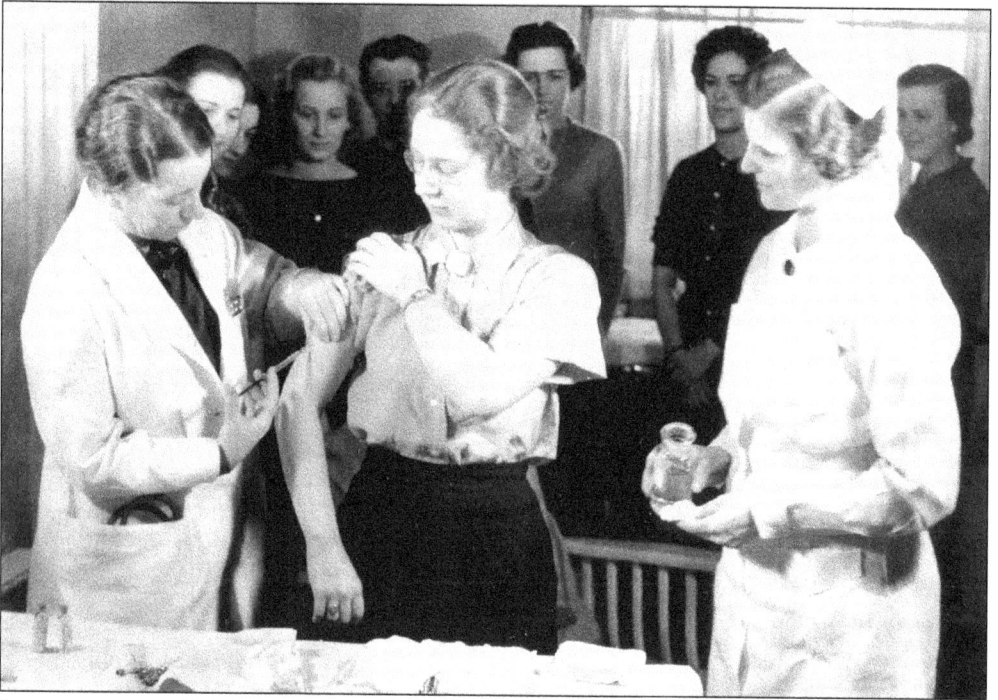

IMMUNIZATIONS. Only young women of excellent health were accepted as students. Every effort was made to keep them healthy. Seen here, Dr. F. Constance Stewart, the physician in charge of health service, is giving an injection, one of the least-attractive aspects of maintaining good health status. The tuberculosis vaccination bacillus Calmette-Guérin (BCG) was often referred to by the students as "the meat stamp" and consisted of more than 40 simultaneous punctures.

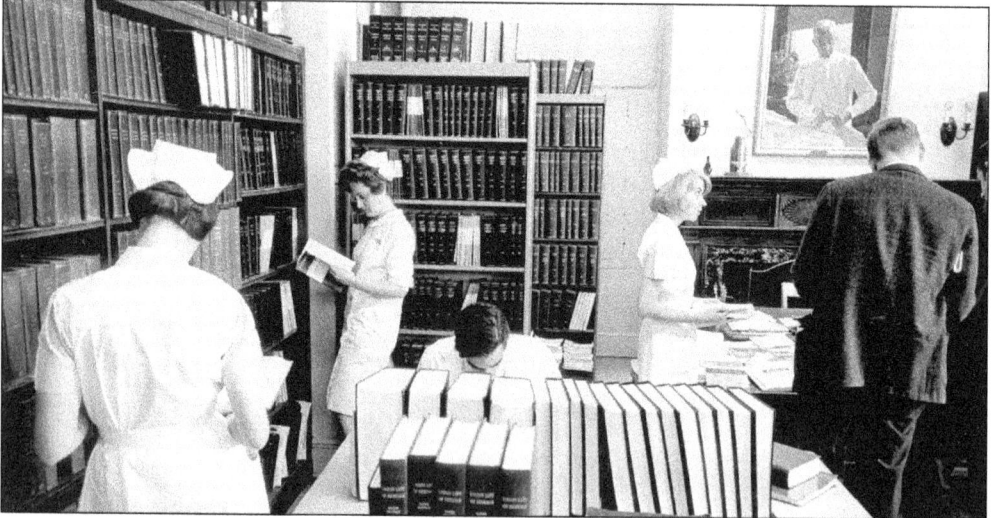

THE ALBANY MEDICAL COLLEGE LIBRARY. The library, which also housed the collection of nursing volumes, was a vital part of the students' education process. Many hours were spent in the reading room located on the first floor of Albany Medical College. The New York State Library was within walking distance and augmented study by an interchange of books and periodicals. The film library was another service of the state library.

PROGRESS REPORTS. At frequent intervals, students had the opportunity to discuss their progress with an adviser from the nursing faculty. The adviser assisted the students by letting them know what they had done well and where efforts were needed for further improvement.

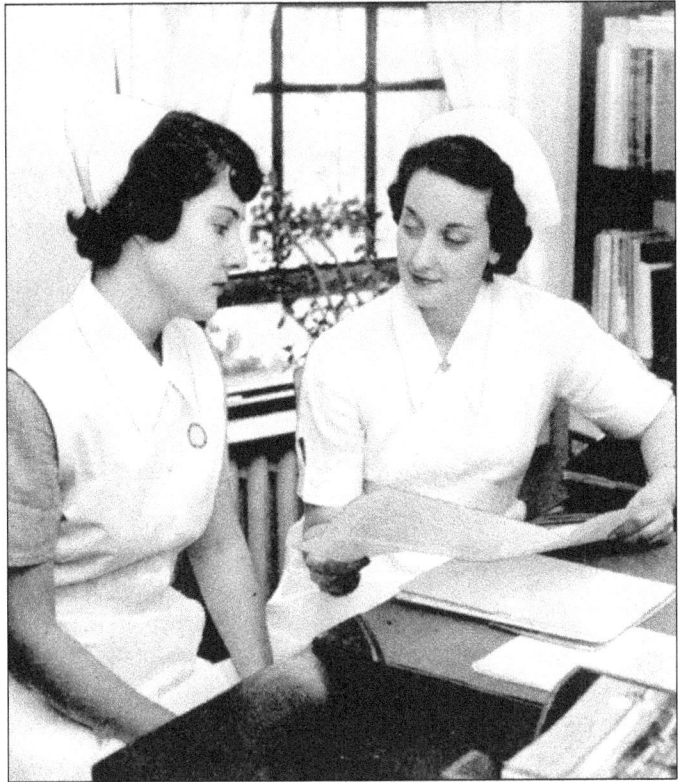

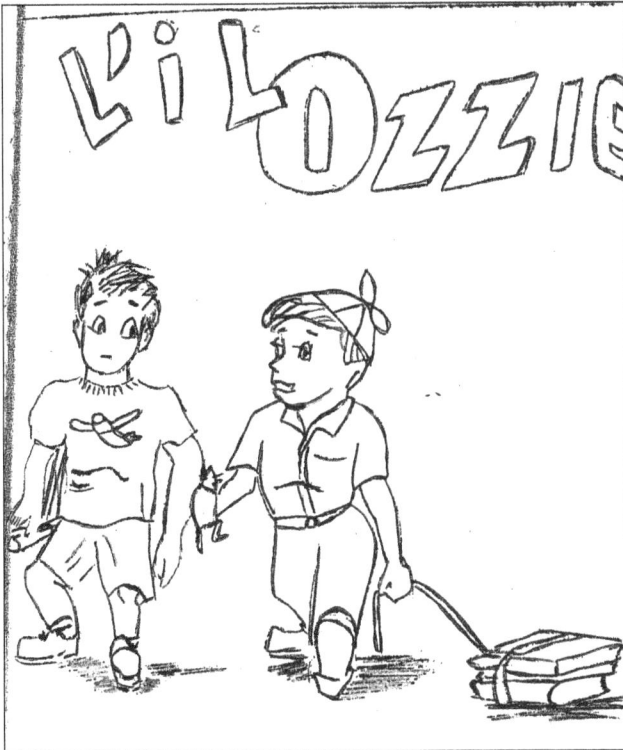

L'IL OZZIE. In this cartoon, L'il Ozzie is telling his friend, "I had the toughest time of my life. First I got Angina Pectoris; then Arteriosclerosis. Just as I was recovering from these, I got Tuberculosis, Pneumonia and Phthisis. They gave me Hypodermics. Appendicitis was followed by Tonsillectomy. I know I had Diabetes and Indigestion, besides Gastritis, Rheumatism and Lumbago. I don't know how I ever pulled through it. It was the hardest spelling test I ever had." (Courtesy *Stethoscope*.)

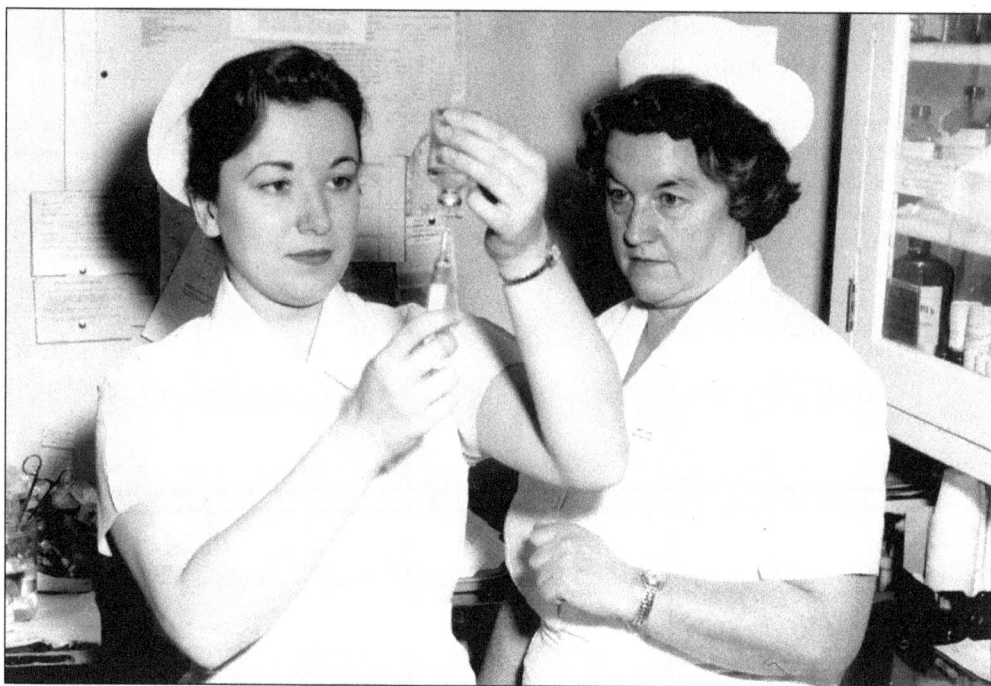

A Nursing Student Supervised on Passing Medications. Passing medications without supervision was a goal of great importance. Accuracy, promptness, and maintaining sterile technique were all to be achieved before a student nurse went solo and received the coveted green dot after her name from pharmacology instructor Gertrude King, R.N., Class of Spring 1948 (see page 74).

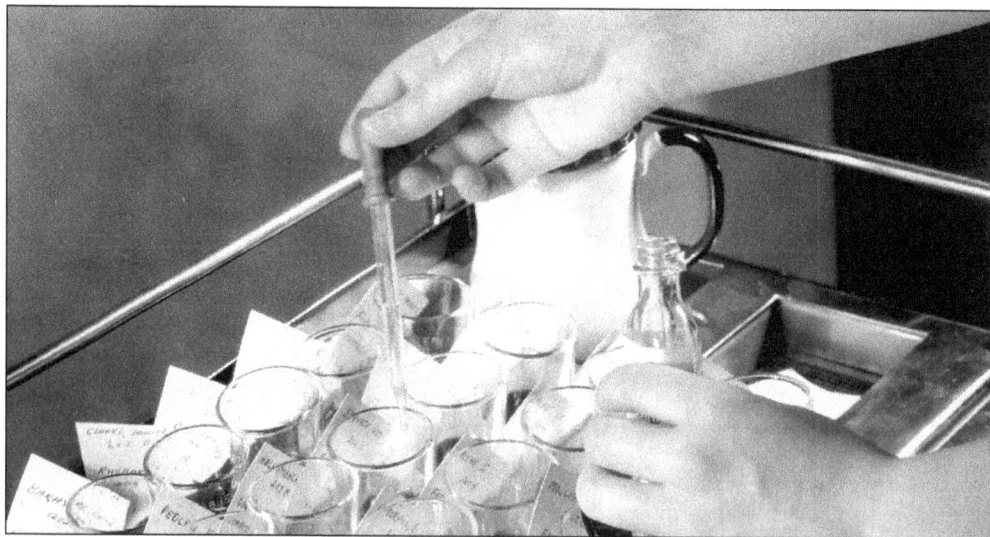

A Medication Nurse. In the 1950s, functional nursing was widely used. World War II dramatically changed the way nurses perceived the profession of nursing. Hospital nursing evolved from private duty to functional method with specific tasks assigned. The medicine nurse gave all medications identified by white tickets and the treatment nurse did nursing procedures denoted by green tickets. Other assignments were giving baths, making beds, and charge duties. Students were assigned to all these responsibilities.

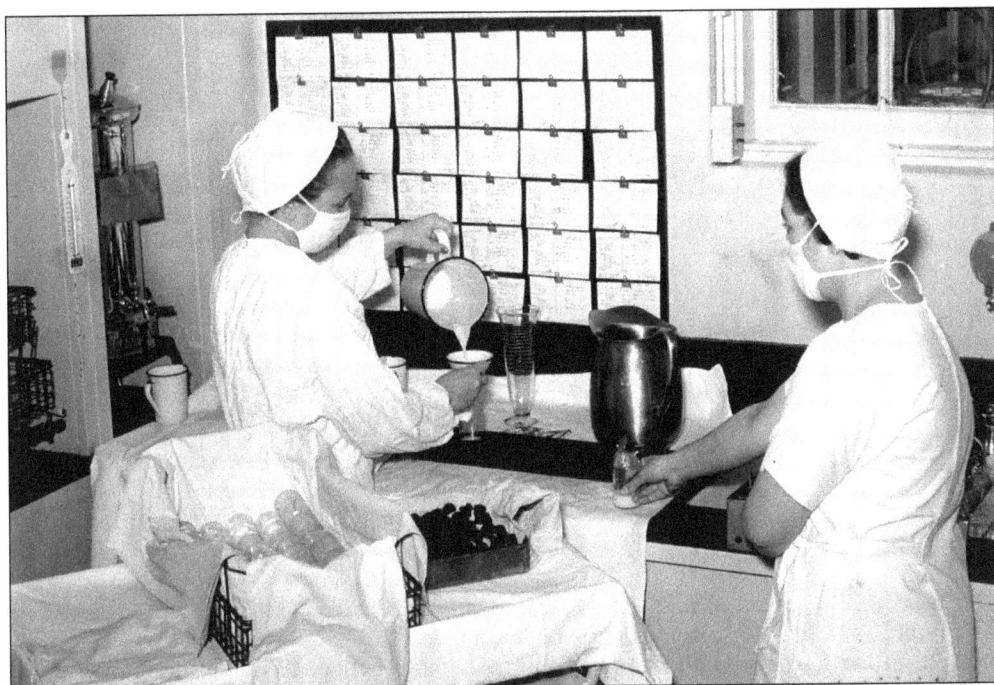

NURSES PREPARE FORMULAS. Nurses were assigned to the formula room, where directions were followed to prepare formulas from scratch for newborns and pediatric patients needing liquid nourishment.

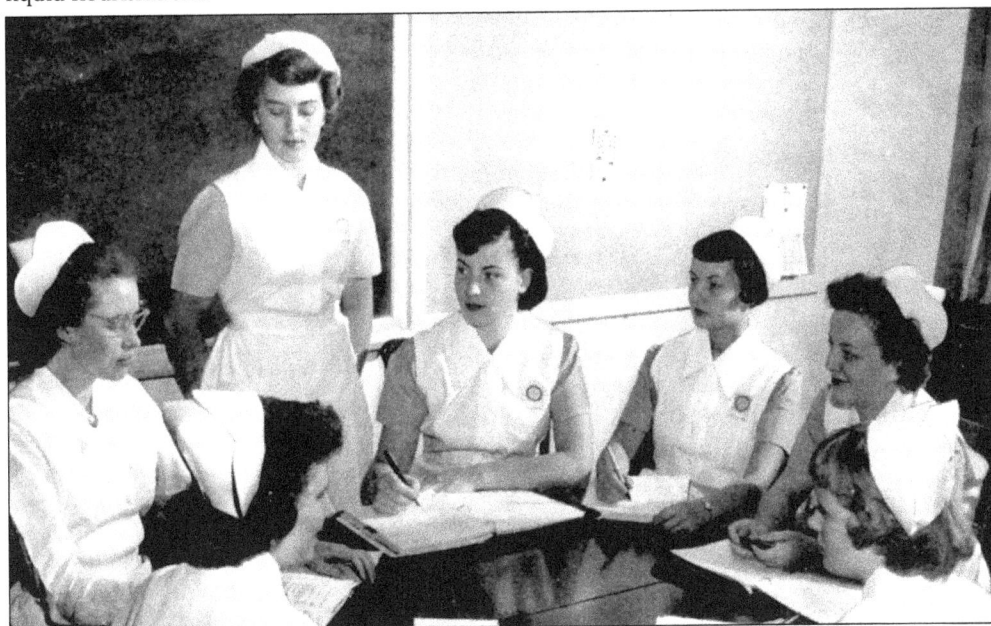

YOUR IDEAS ARE IMPORTANT. Participation in group discussions was encouraged. To present input in a clear and objective manner contributed to group decisions, with each student having a part in its formation. A positive byproduct was the personal growth of the student. Student uniforms, jumpers with the Union University logo and checked-sleeve blouses, are apparent. The UUSN cap with three scallops denoted that, until then, there were three nursing schools.

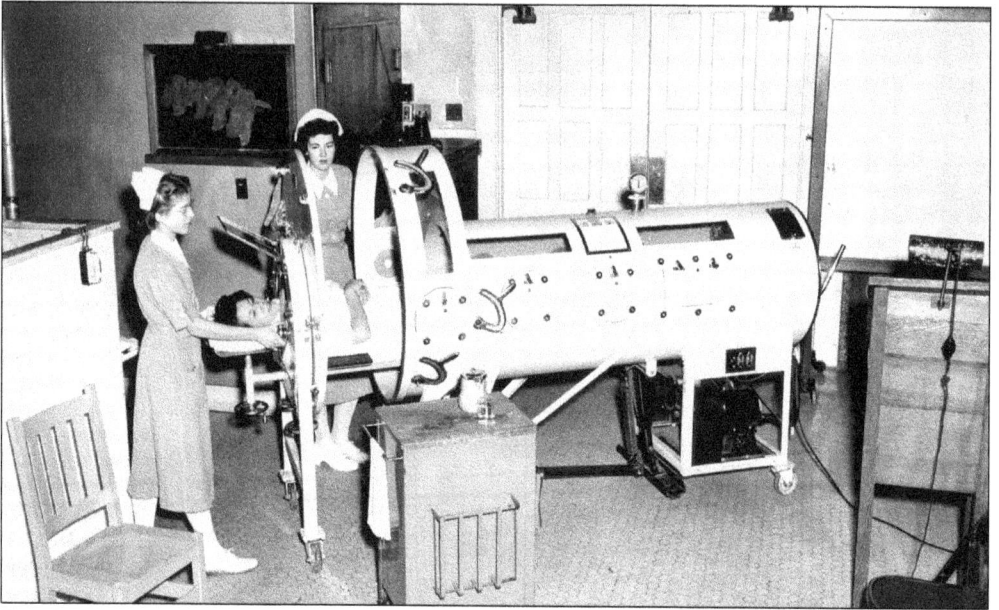

THE IRON LUNG. Iron lungs stored on the ramp connecting the nurses' residence to the hospital were all in use for patients during the polio epidemics of the 1940s and 1950s. Emergency care instruction included how to use the hand pump at the end of the iron lung to maintain a patient's respirations in case of a power failure. Albany Hospital was the first polio center in upstate New York.

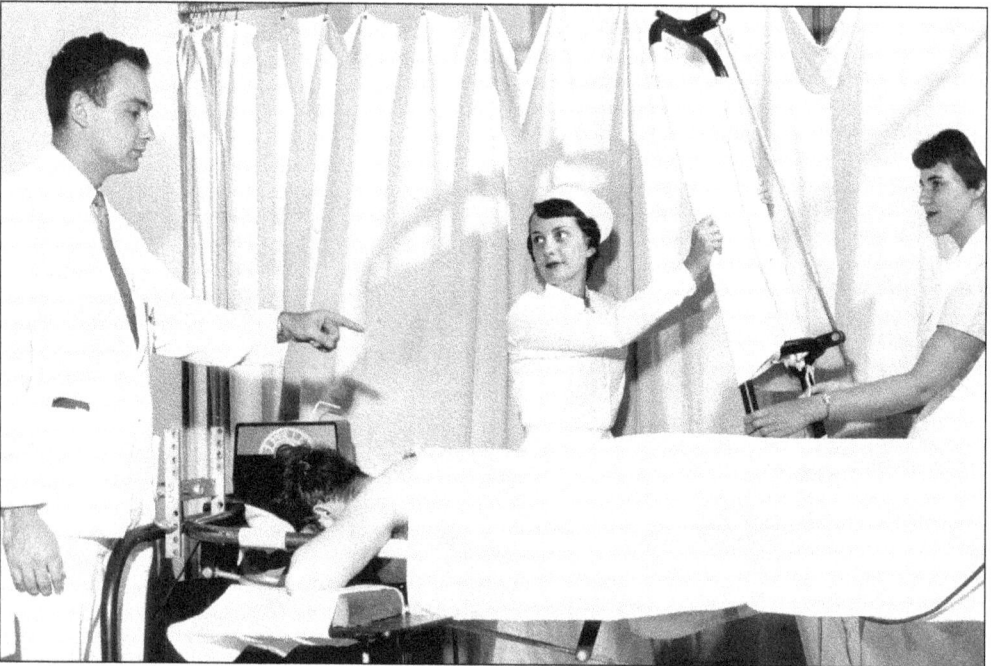

A STRYKER FRAME PROCEDURE. Instructor Grace Druzba Pugliese, R.N., Class of 1954, and a student receive a pointer from the intern as they apply the top part of the Stryker frame to turn a patient from facedown to faceup. The Stryker frame was used for patients with paralysis or those needing to remain immobile to prevent bed sores and pneumonia.

TRANSPORTATION VIA WHEELCHAIR. Students were often the means of transporting patients to tests, other departments, or on a recreational jaunt to the outside roof, lobby, or lounge. This task is now assigned to the transportation department. Note the design of the wheelchair.

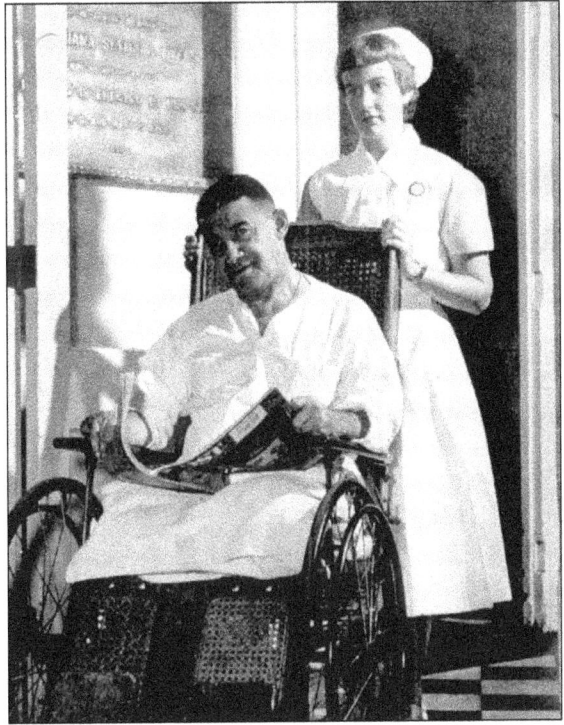

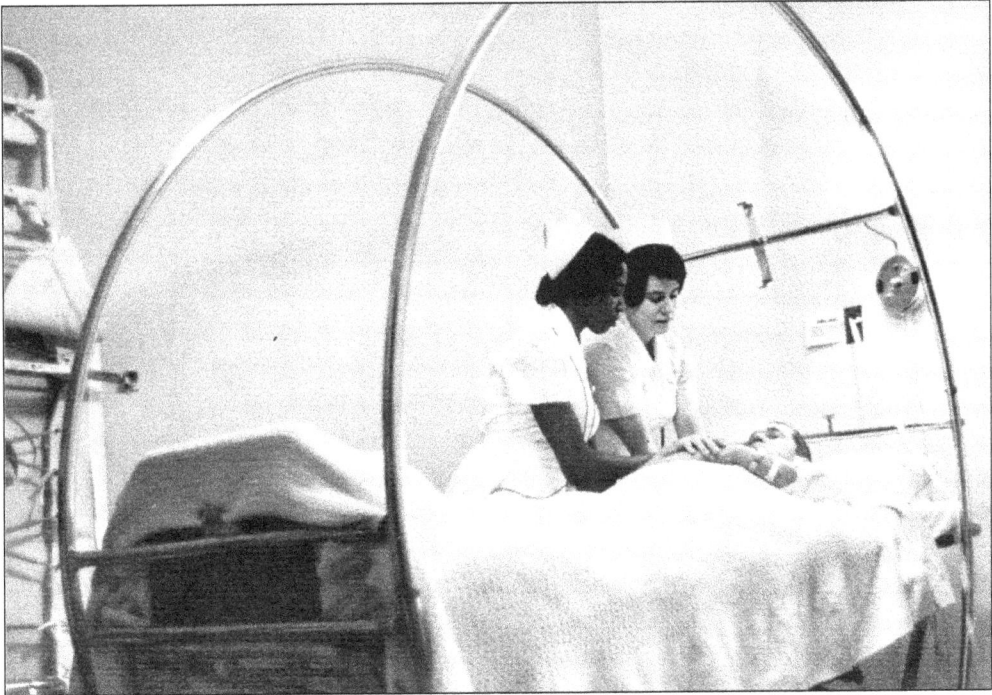

THE ROCKING BED. The use of the rocking bed had advantages over the Stryker frame. It was a wider bed that rotated the patient from a lying position to an upright position and back again. This enabled the patient to breathe easier and prevented secretions from settling in the lungs, causing hypostatic pneumonia.

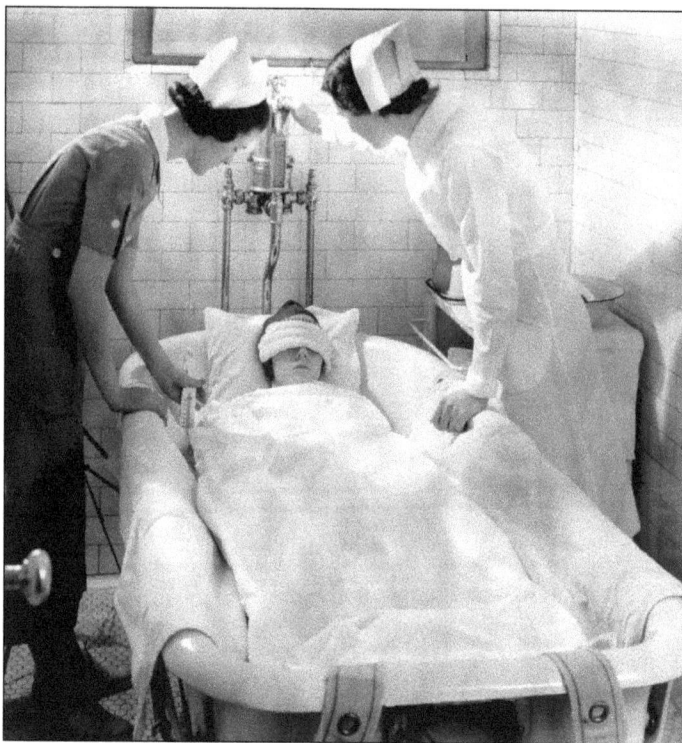

HYDROTHERAPY. This therapy was used as a sedative for patients with nervous and mental disorders. The nurses shown here are checking the temperature of the water.

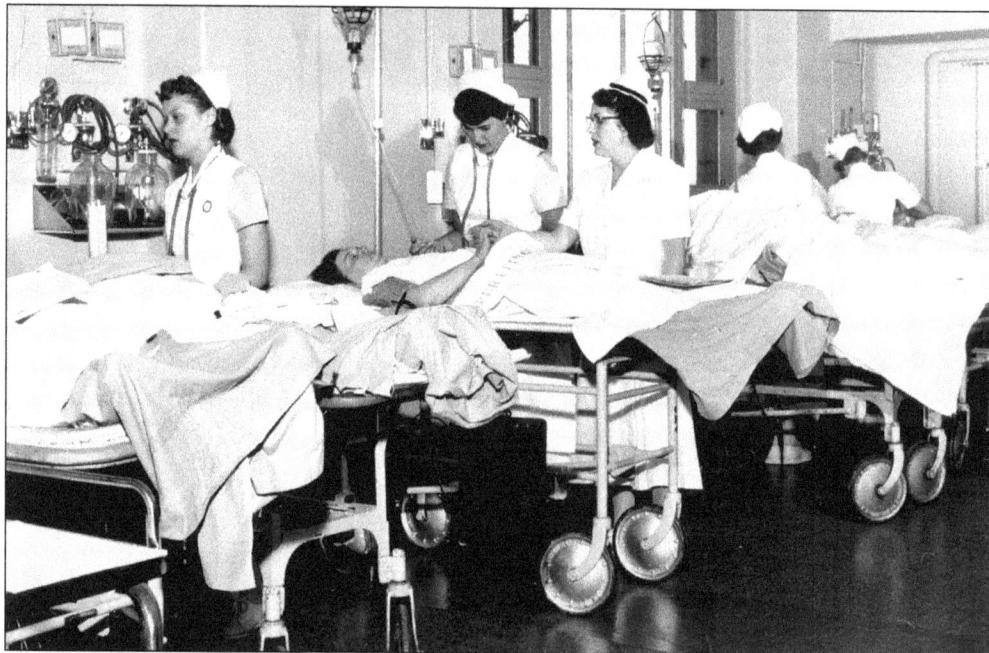

THE RECOVERY ROOM. It was a boon to nurses to have surgical patients side by side in the new recovery room (*c.* 1952). Nurses did not have to run from patients' rooms at one end of the corridor to the other to check vital signs every 15 minutes. Patients could also be more closely supervised until they regained consciousness and the danger of bleeding had decreased. In 1953, recovery room experience was added in medical and surgical nursing.

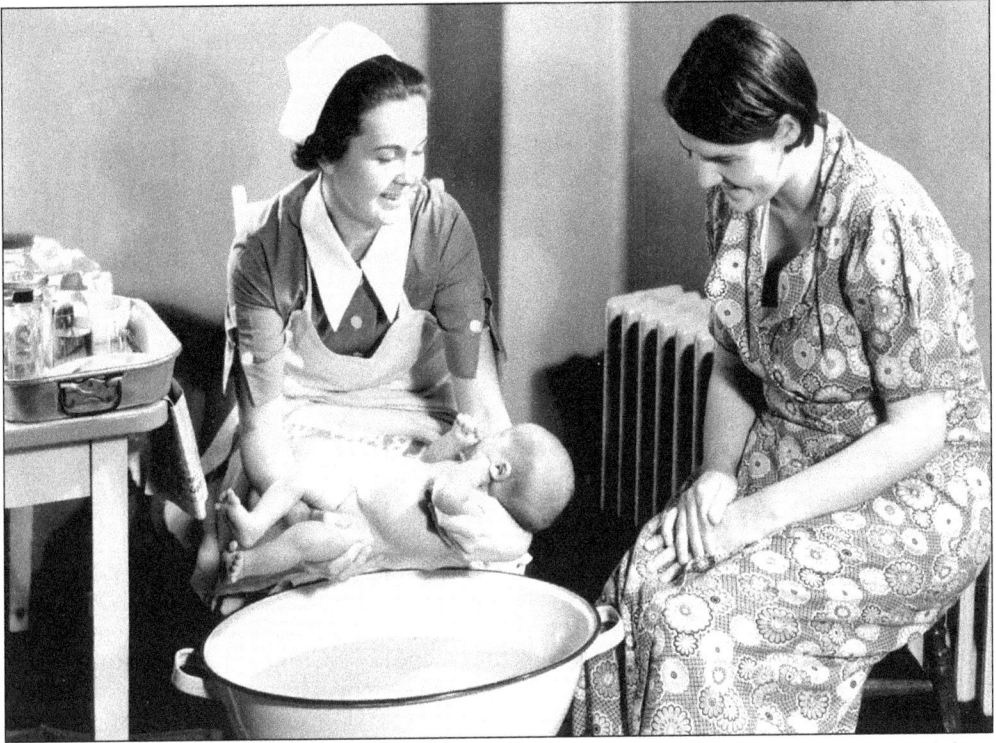

VISITING NURSING. Senior RSCSN and UUSN students had visiting nursing as part of their curriculum. In 1954, it became an elective for UUSN students. Newspapers were used to cover work areas and, as seen in the photograph, they were folded and used as bags for unwanted material. Who is going to get the wettest when the baby starts to kick? Home nursing involved care of sick, teaching healthcare measures, newborn care, and referrals to community resources.

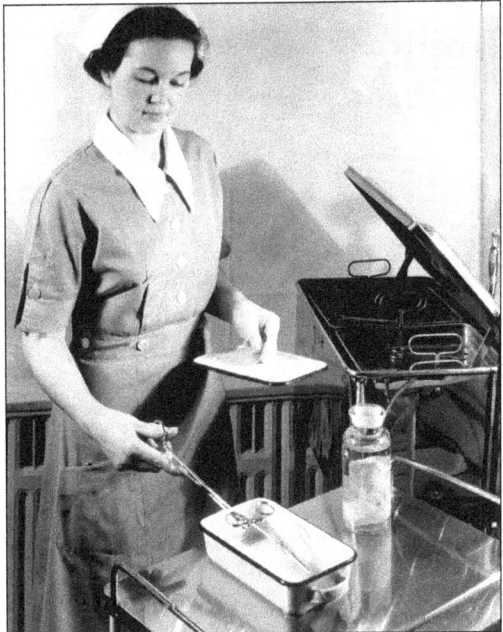

A BOILING WATER STERILIZER. A supply of instruments was kept on the ward for changing dressings and was sterilized between uses. Forceps kept in disinfecting solution were used to lift the instruments from the sterilizer. Packaged supplies sterilized by autoclaving came from central supply, the delivery room, and the operating room.

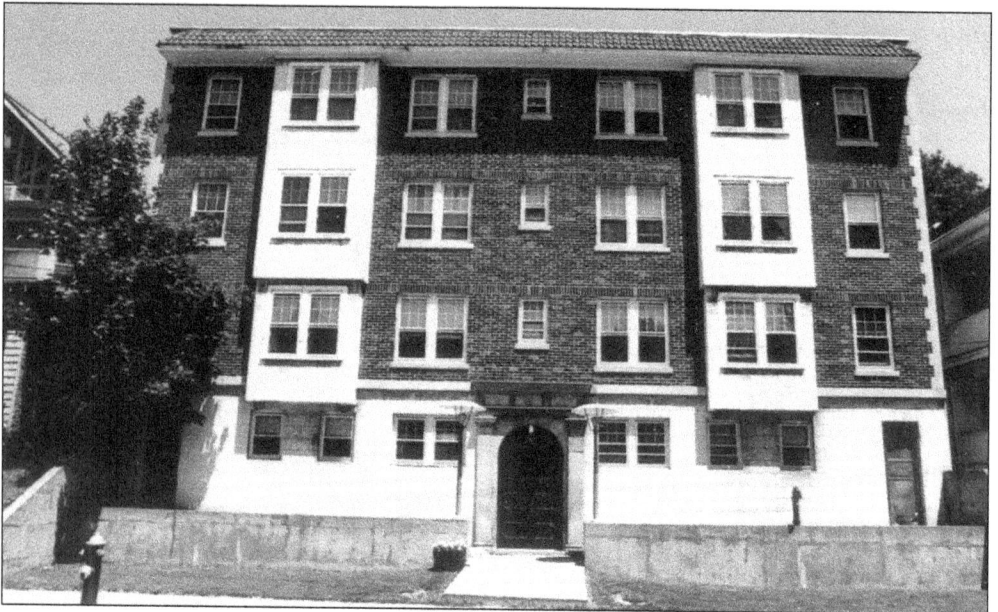

MORRIS HALL. Morris Hall was an apartment house located about three blocks from Albany Hospital. In students' second and third years, they moved to apartment living from the single room arrangement of the "old Residence." There was a communal living room for the residence, and each apartment had a kitchenette. Security escort service was provided for students on evening and night duty assignments.

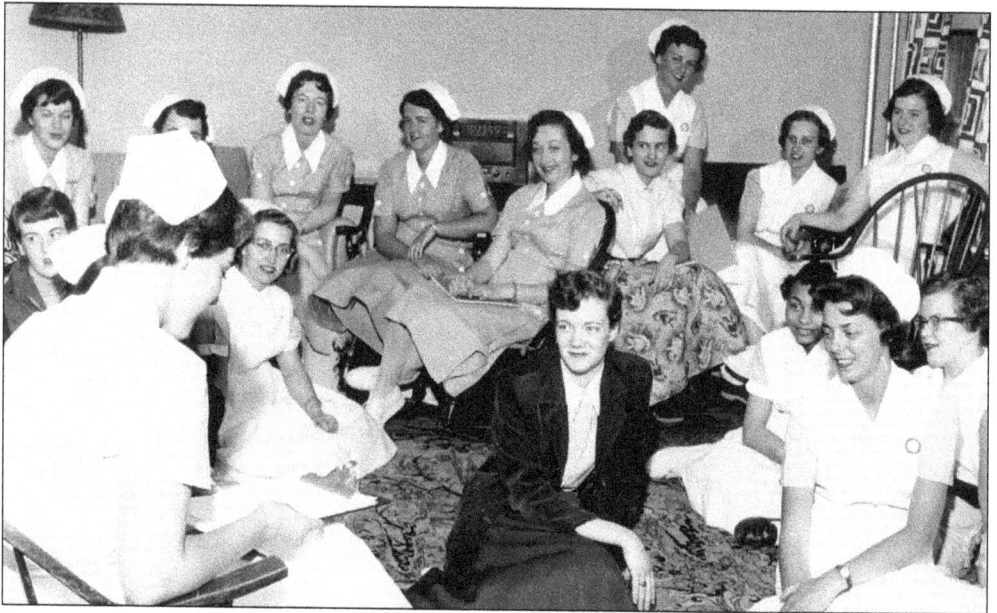

STUDENT GOVERNMENT. Students from four schools are represented on student council. The schools represented were RSCSN, UUSN, Plattsburgh (see page 63), and, seated in the chair, AMCSN, the newcomer. Student self-government promoted an understanding of the democratic principles of group living, developed leadership initiatives, and promoted an appreciation of cooperative methods of problem solving. The faculty adviser assisted as a liaison between faculty and students.

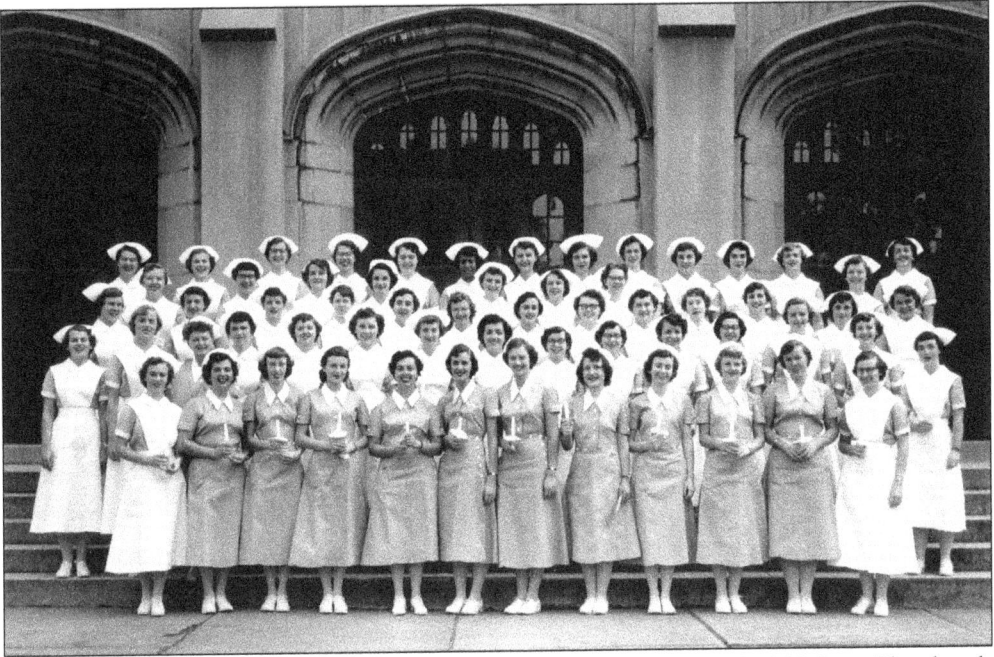

NURSING SCHOOLS AFFILIATED AT UUSN. Students in the Class of 1955 from Plattsburgh State Teachers College (PSTC), division of School Nurse-Teacher Education, flank the RSCSN students immediately following their capping ceremony. Students from these three schools had the same scientific and clinical curriculum while at the hospital. (Courtesy Janet Zubinski Tuomey.)

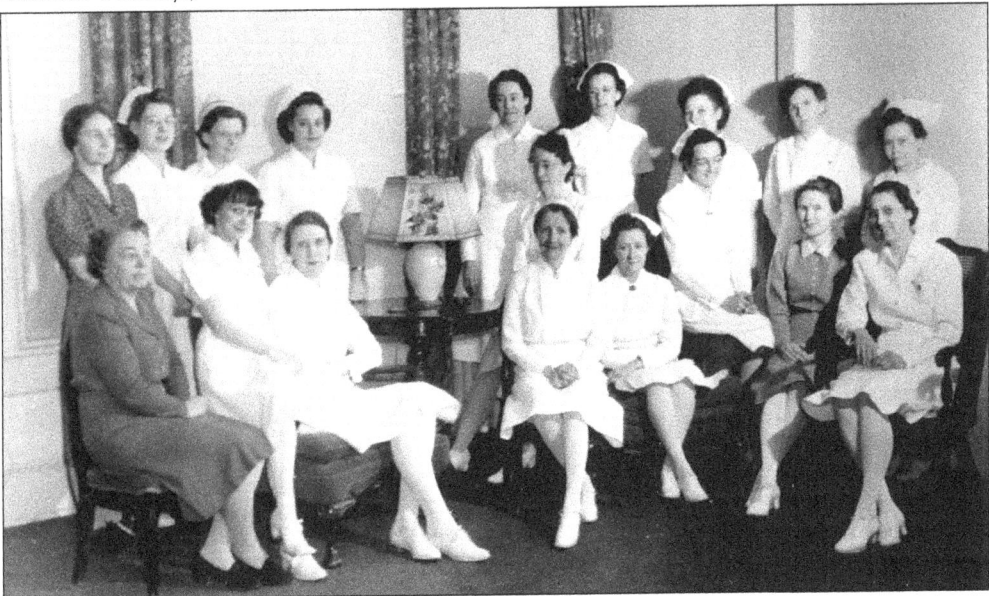

RSCSN FACULTY. Faculty members of the college who taught clinical subjects were closely connected with the hospital. Two directors of RSCSN became directors of UUSN. Elizabeth A. Bell (front row, second from the right) was director of RSCSN from 1944 to 1947 and UUSN from 1944 to 1947. Mildred C. Boeke (front row, third from the left) was director of RSCSN from 1947 to 1948 and director of UUSN from 1947 to 1952.

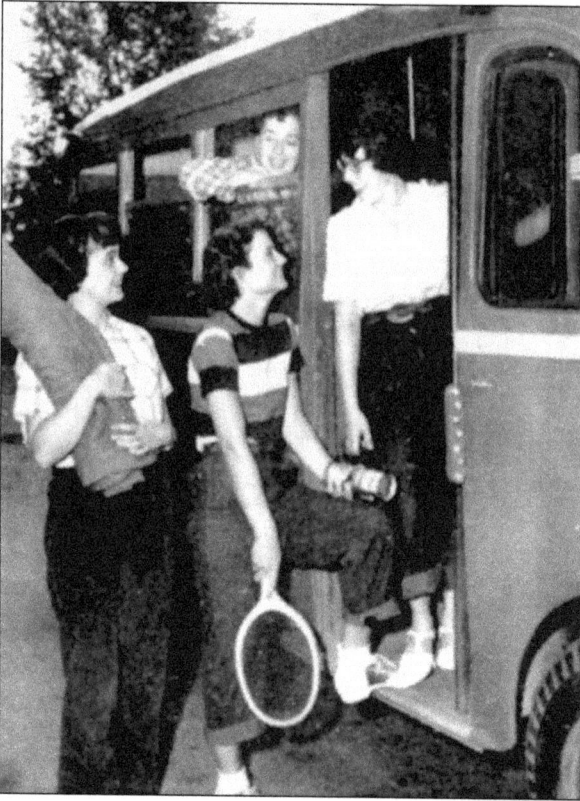

A LEADERSHIP CONFERENCE
OR SCHOOL PICNIC. Leadership
conference was a day away
for old and new student
government officers to evaluate
past endeavors and plan new
ones. The school picnic was a
day of fun, games, and food for
all the students not on duty.

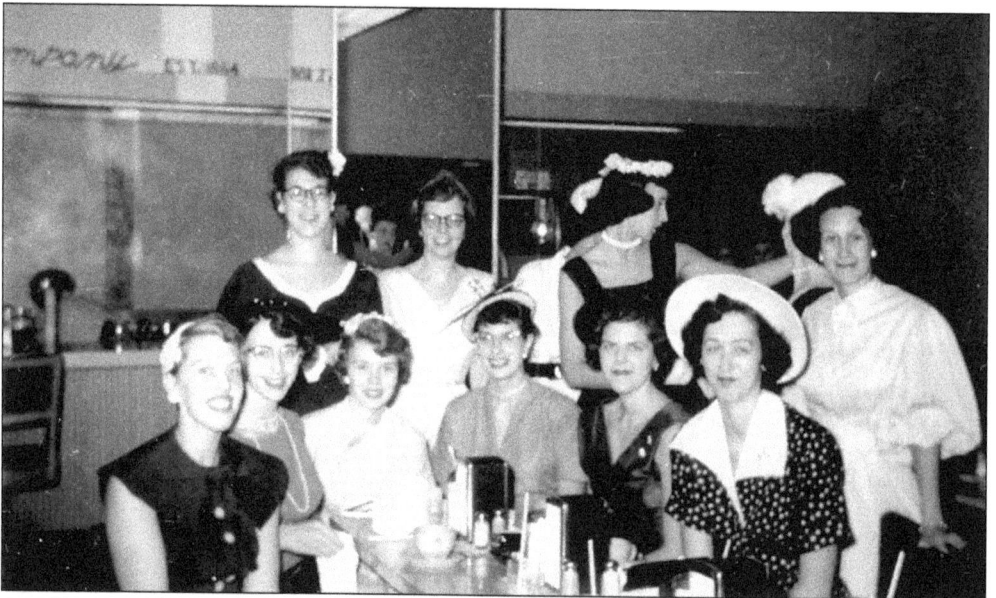

ALL DRESSED UP FOR BACCALAUREATE SERVICE. UUSN students in the Class of 1955 are all
dressed up at a time when hats were a must to attend the graduation baccalaureate service.
Seen here are, from left to right, the following: (front row) Elaine Goodrich, Florence Dunning,
Janet Buchanan, Eina Conde, Jessica Pendt, and Marjorie Sheley; (back row) Jane Savage, Joan
Vrooman, Betty Ann Santas, and Shirley Swartz. (Courtesy Joan Vrooman Mitchell, R.N.)

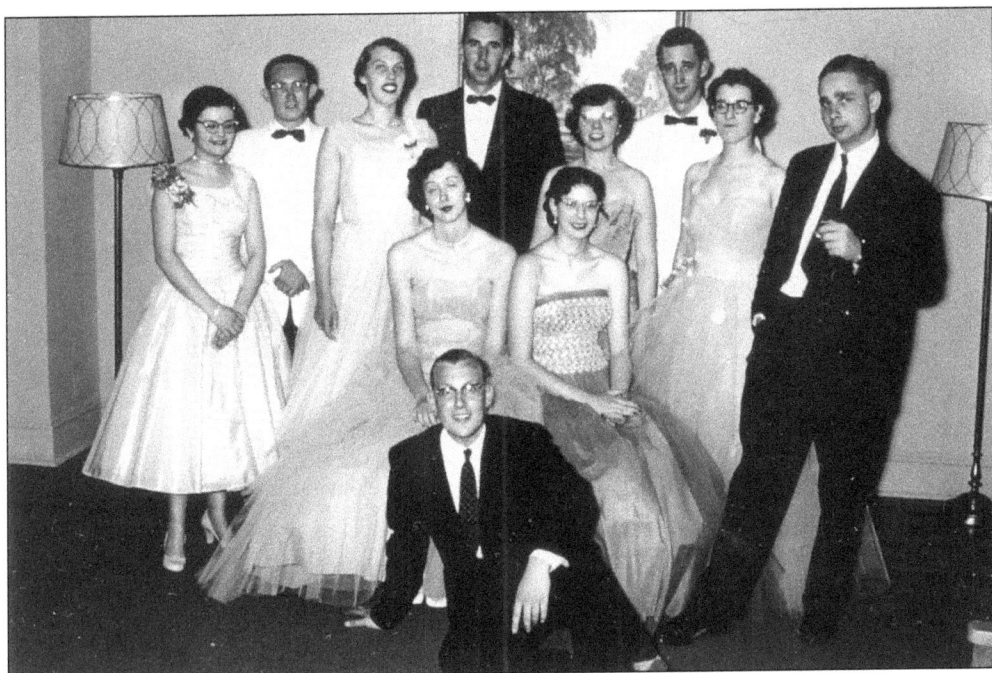

OH, HOW WE'LL DANCE! Couples pose for a 1955 senior ball photograph. The women standing are, from left to right, Jean Biscotti, Elaine Goodrich, Joan Vrooman, and Jane Savage. The women sitting are Marjorie Sheley (left) and Eina Conde (right). (Courtesy Eina O'Day.)

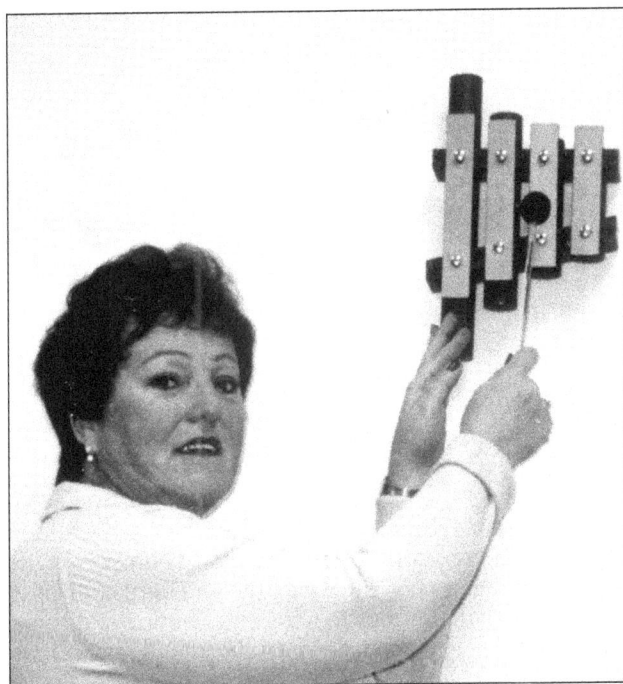

THE WARD GONG, AN EARLY VERSION OF THE BEEPER. Paula Zenzen, R.N., Class of Spring 1966, who rescued this gong from the demolition crew, shows its use when functional assignments were popular. One gong called the charge nurse, two gongs called the medicine nurse, and three gongs called the treatment nurse. A gift to the Alumni Association, it will be mounted with the permanent nursing exhibit off the Pillars Lobby.

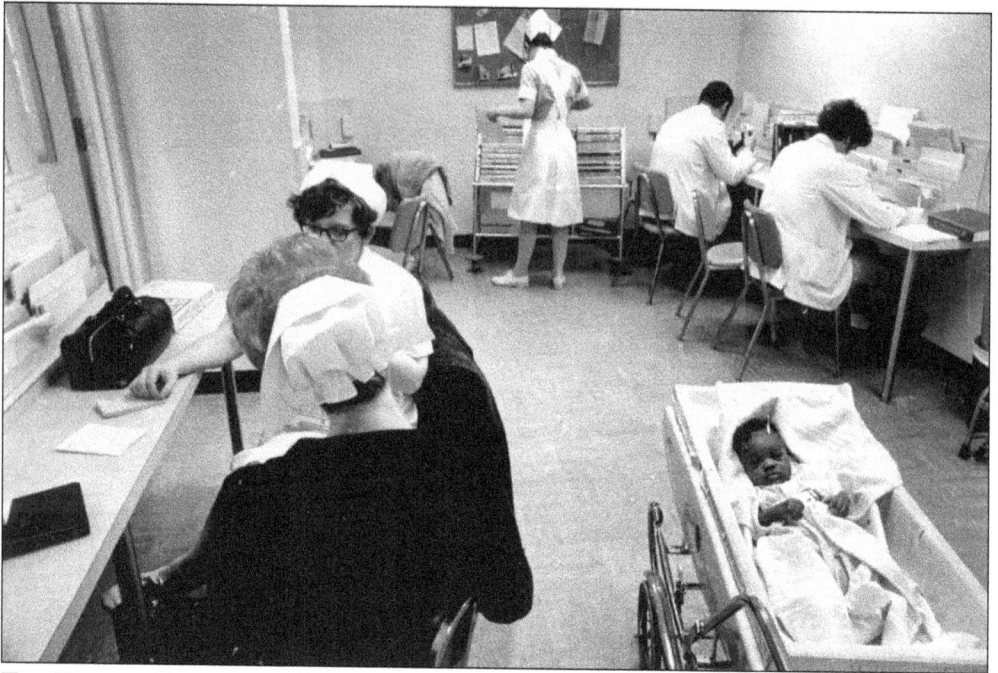

THE NURSING STATION. Staff nurses, an instructor, a student, interns, and the little patient in the carriage are all part of the interaction at the pediatrics nursing station. Staff members would sometimes bring patients to the nursing station so they could complete other duties, such as charting, team conferences, and change-of-shift report.

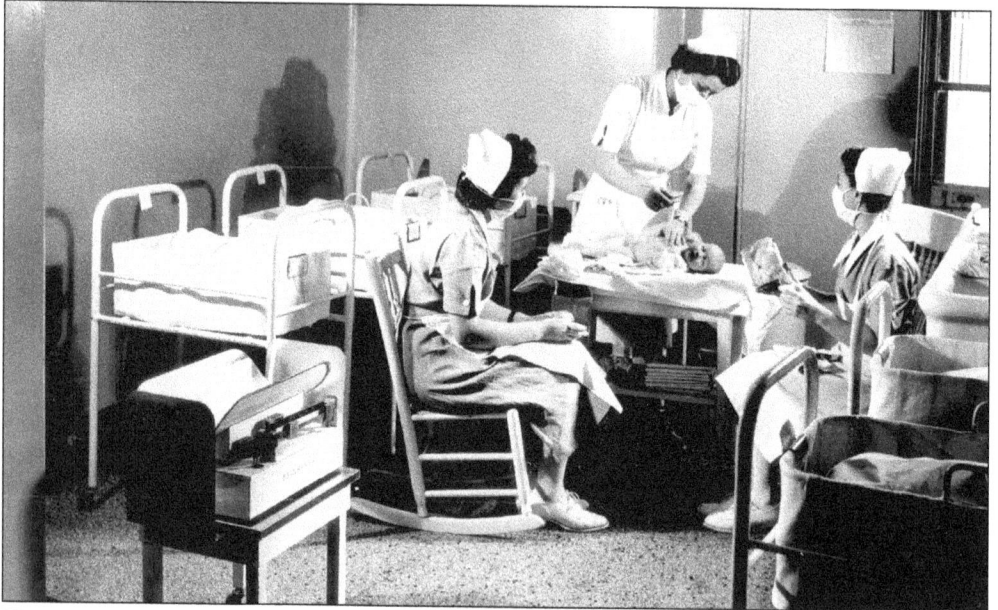

HANDS-ON INSTRUCTION IN THE NEWBORN NURSERY. Checking the newborn during the bath was a good time to note how well the umbilical cord and circumcision areas were healing. A bath was more than a time for cleansing. Noting skin condition and coloration, breath sounds, and body range of motion, as well as bonding responses, were important observations. Nursing students also taught mothers newborn care on a baby mannequin.

AN ALBANY HOSPITAL BILL. Before bills were typed or computer generated, they were completed by hand. Look at the seven-day charges for hospital care of the mother in 1949. A separate bill shows that seven days of room and board for the baby was $7. (Courtesy Donald H. Miller.)

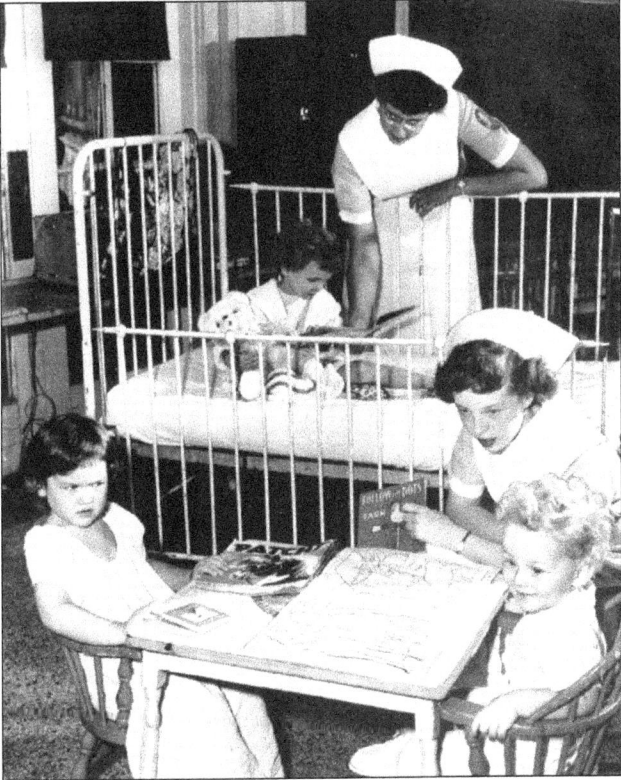

PEDIATRIC CLINICAL EXPERIENCE. Morning care is complete, and now it is time for play. PSTCSN students have two happy campers and one who is not so sure. What will the instructor say about the crib side being down and the student being on the other side of the crib?

67

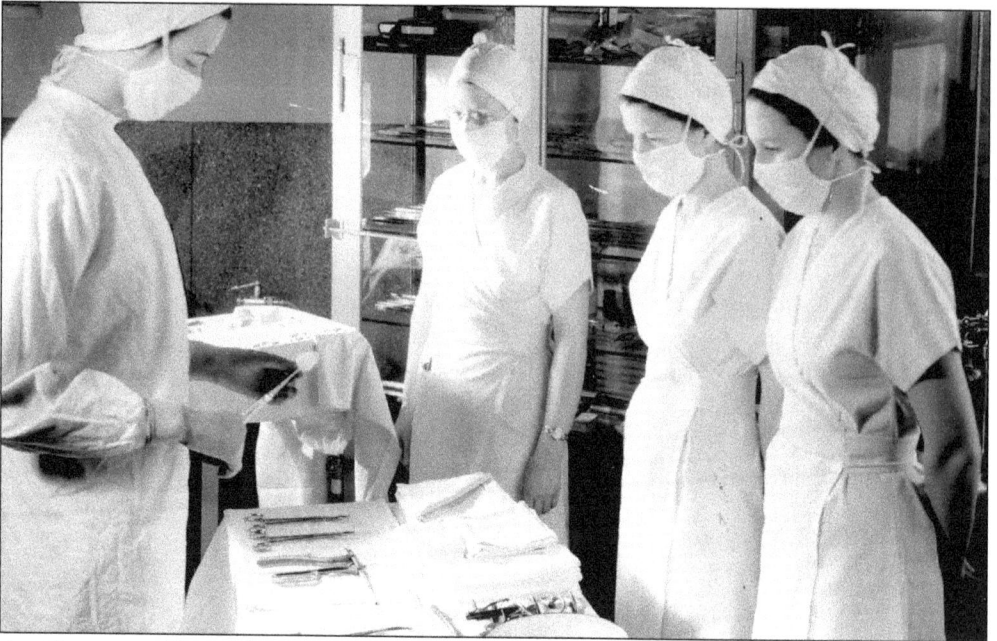

AN OPERATING ROOM SCRUB CLASS. When assigned to the operating room, students learned the names of each instrument, where they were placed on the table, how they were handed to the surgeon, and, above all, how to maintain a sterile field. An important aside was to know what the surgeon called the instrument he wanted. The practice session was a breeze.

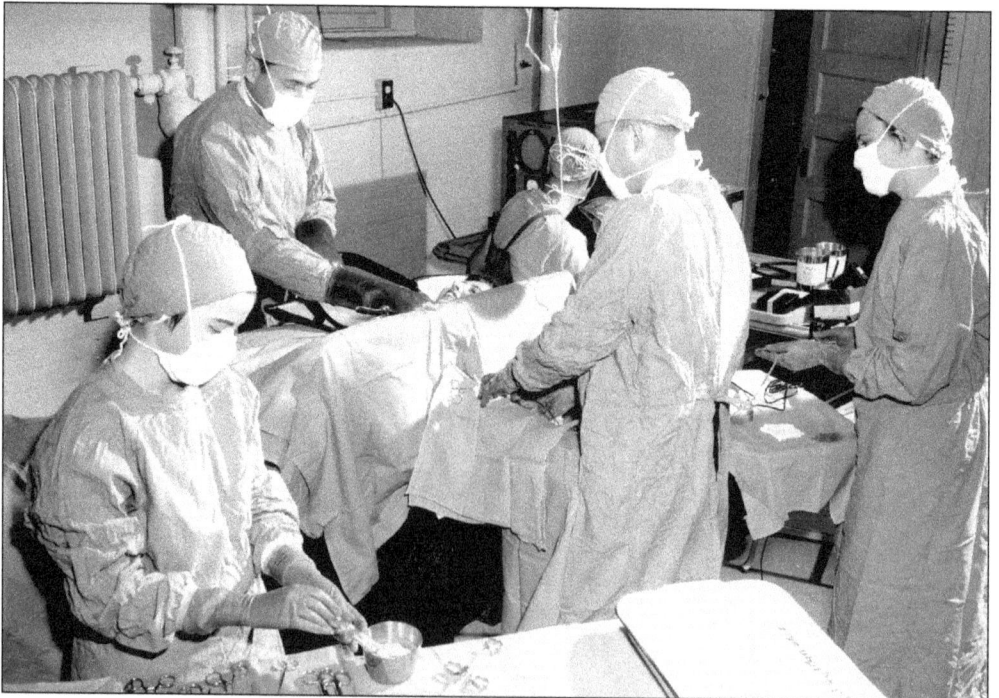

AN OPERATING ROOM SCRUB NURSE. This student has reason to be nervous, as it is her first time as a scrub nurse. It is a matter of record that student scrub nurses were discharged from a case if they handed the surgeon the incorrect instrument.

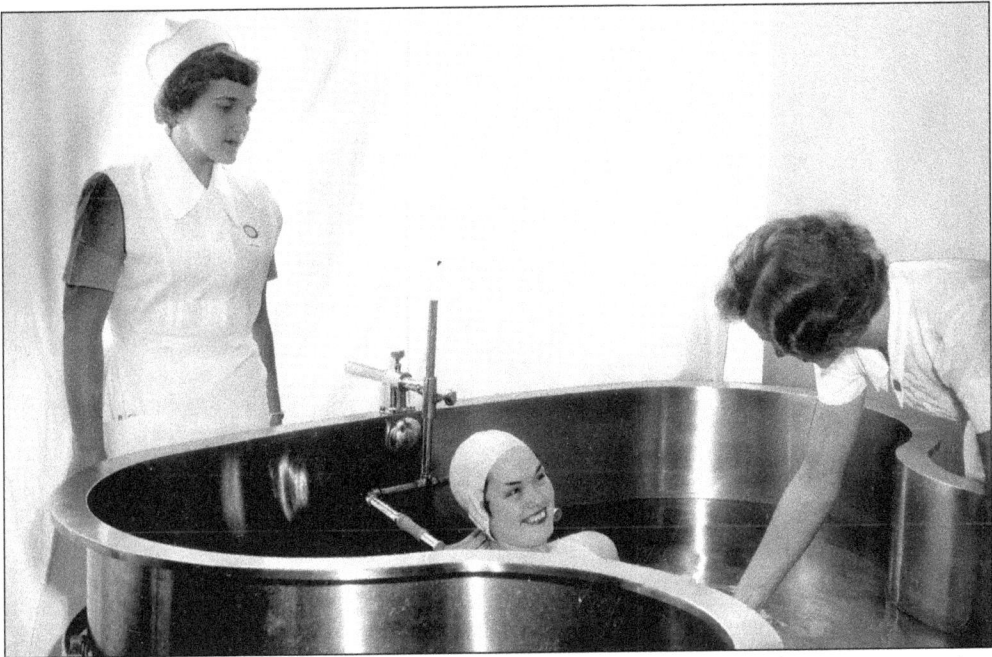

PHYSICAL THERAPY. Students would often accompany patients to tests and treatments in other departments to gain a greater understanding of the total care a patient was receiving. Pictured are a UUSN student and a therapist administering hydrotherapy to a patient in the physical therapy department.

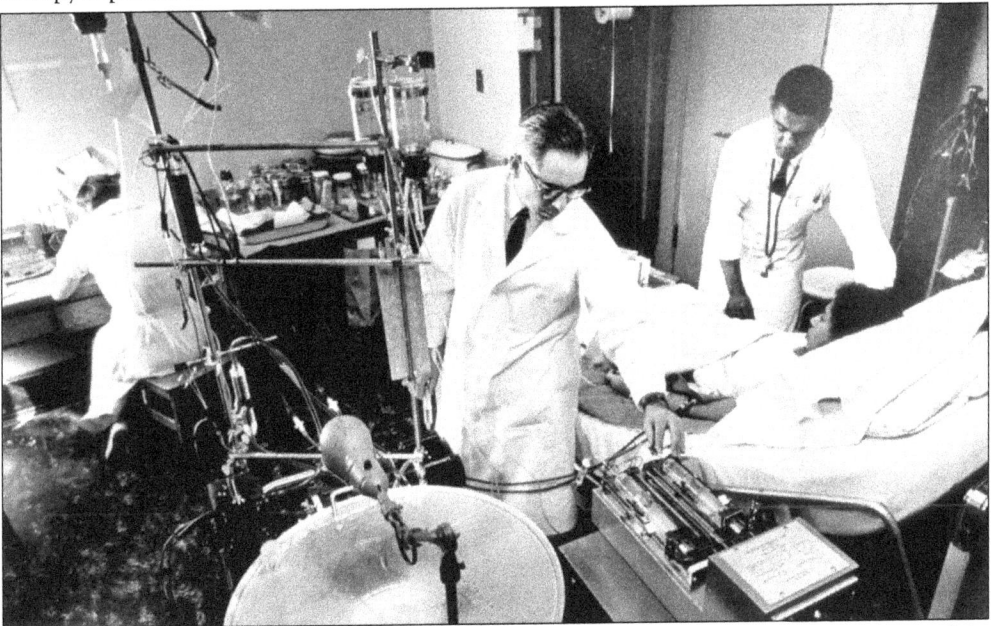

AN ARTIFICIAL KIDNEY. The hospital was one of five institutions to have this innovative life-saving device in 1950. Performing dialysis are Dr. William Kiley (left) and Dr. Orlando Hines. Senior nurses were assigned to assist the physician in this intricate procedure. The size of the original artificial kidney machine required a single-sized bedroom to operate. A bedroom on the third floor of the nurses' residence was chosen.

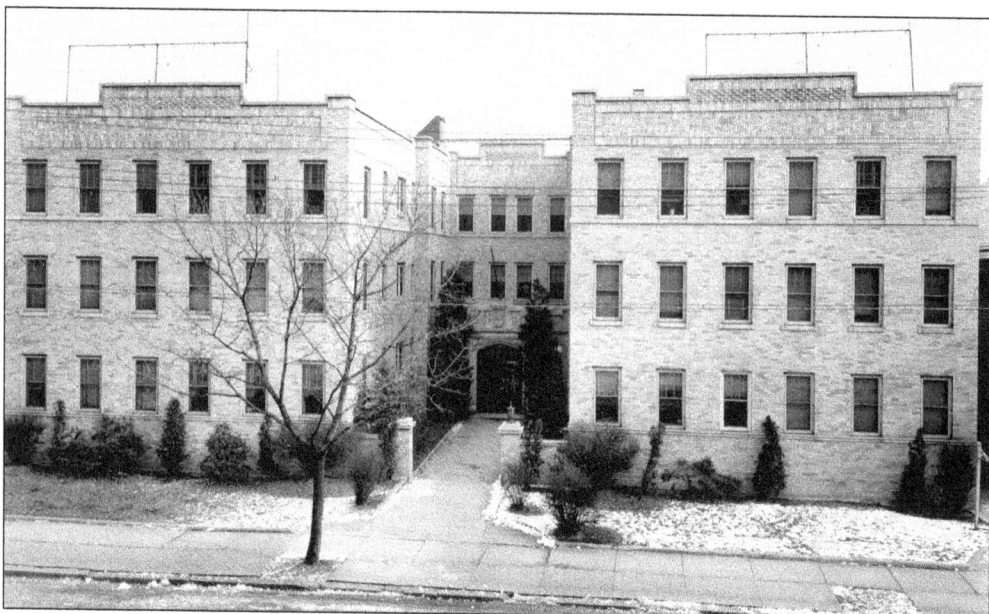

BOLTON HALL. RSCSN and Albany Hospital participated jointly in the U.S. Cadet Nurse Corps, which trained nurses during the war from 1943 until recruitment terminated in September 1945. The newly acquired nurses' residence, Bolton Hall, was named in honor of Frances Payne-Bolton, who spearheaded the establishment of the nurse corps. Cadets received free tuition, maintenance, uniforms, and a $15 to $30 stipend per month and agreed to serve in emergency civilian jobs or the armed forces.

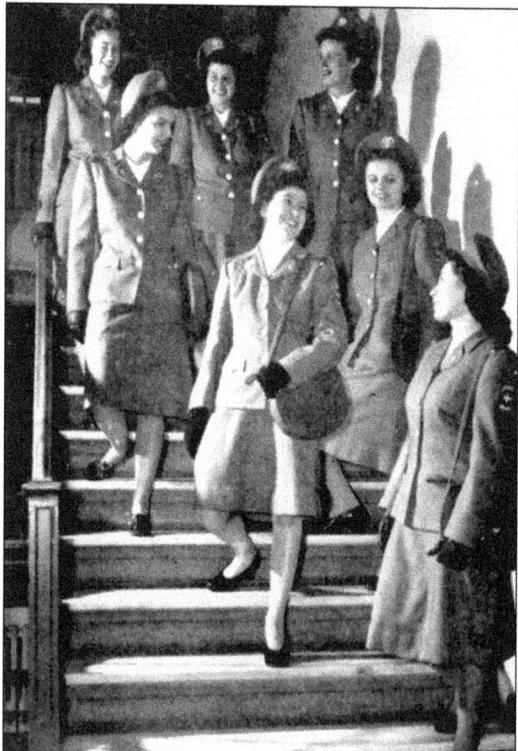

CADETS ON PARADE. Catherine (spelled Katherine in some records) Fee, Class of 1947, wrote the following verse:

Cadets of 1947, passing by.
Cadets of 1947, colors high.
When you see the gray and red beret
   upon our heads,
You'll know when you hear this
   marching song.

Cadets of 1947, in review.
Future nurses of the Army; Navy, too.
And when they write the roll of fame,
You will find the Nurse Corps name,
On the top!

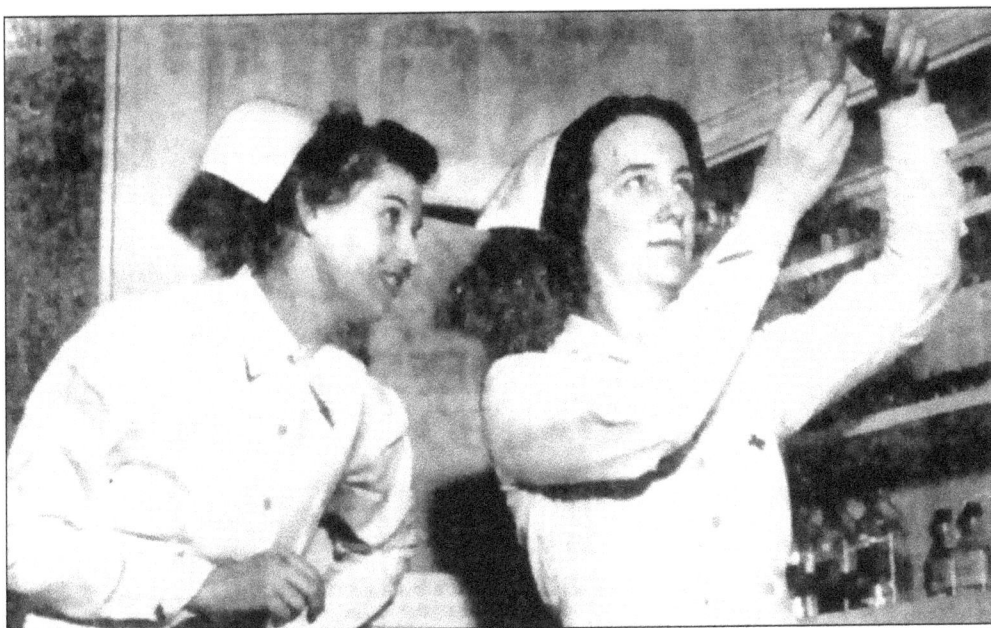

A Refresher Course to Relieve Extreme Shortage. Jacoba Prins Applebee, R.N., an instructor at RSCSN, supervises Helen Ehle as she pours medications in the refresher course at Albany Hospital for nurses inactive for 5 to 15 years. They would then be ready to rejoin the staff as the intensified war effort depleted the nursing staff. (Courtesy *Times Union*, December 28, 1941.)

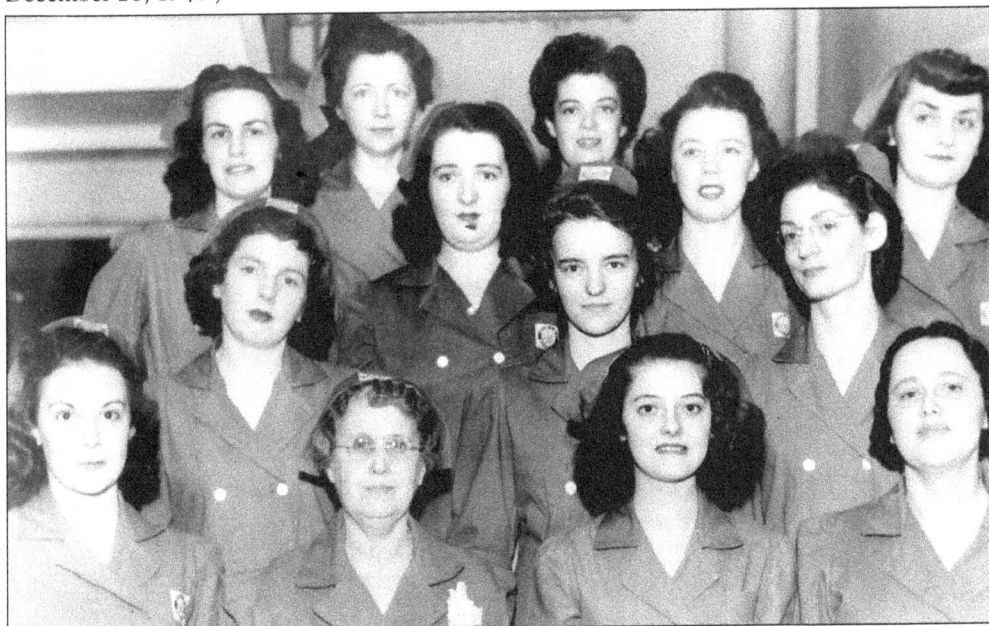

Red Caps. The first evening class of 13 advanced volunteer aides, known as Red Caps, received its colorful blue and red caps on January 5, 1945, prior to being assigned to bathing patients, making beds, and taking temperatures, pulses, and respirations. There were 226 other volunteer aides who worked 3,500 hours in December 1944 without compensation as a patriotic gesture in the war emergency.

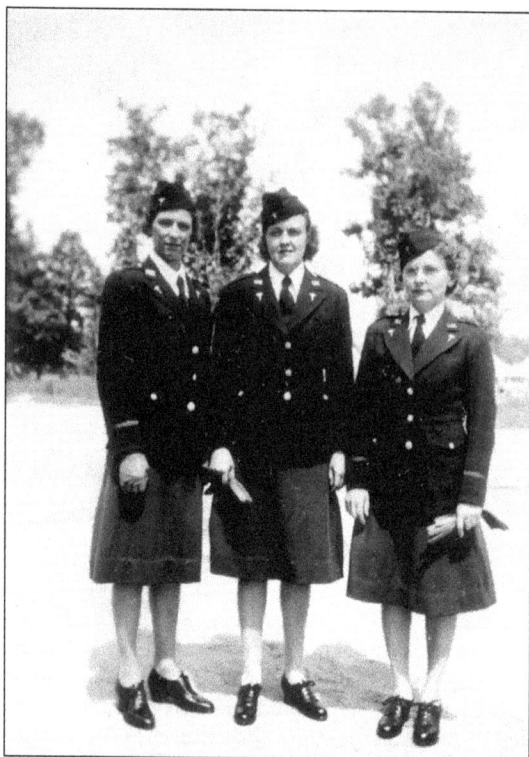

THREE **AHTSN** GRADUATES IN THE ARMY NURSE CORPS. An unidentified nurse (left), Zelda Smith (center), and ? Hagadorn, members of the Class of 1933, were among the 120 area nurses who left for camp on July 15, 1942. The 33rd General Hospital was organized as a 1,000-bed military hospital and cut the Albany Hospital staff by 51 percent. Lt. Col. Eldridge Campbell, attending neurosurgeon, was appointed unit director, and Lt. Col. Richard Beebe was appointed chief of medical services. (Courtesy Daisey Place.)

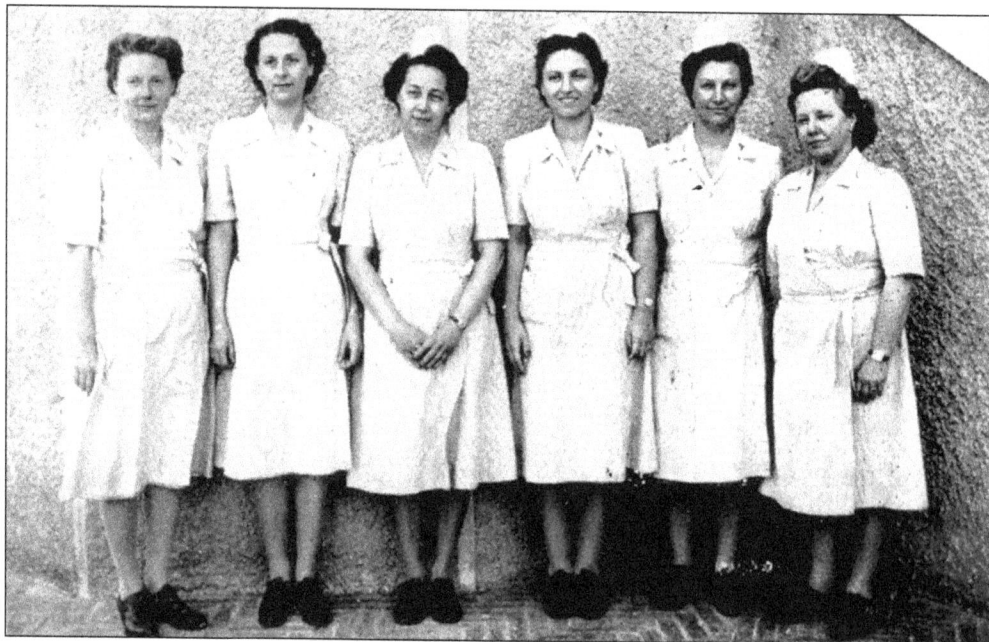

THE CHIEF NURSE, LT. COL. ALICE SPELLMAN, AND OFFICERS. Third from the left, Alice Spellman, R.N., a professor at RSCSN, was chief nurse. She was promoted from first lieutenant to lieutenant colonel. The 1943 annual report noted, "A shower was welcomed after two weeks of using one helmet or less of water a day to keep clean. Cleaned out bullet shells were salvaged to use as connecting tubes for rubber tubing."

72

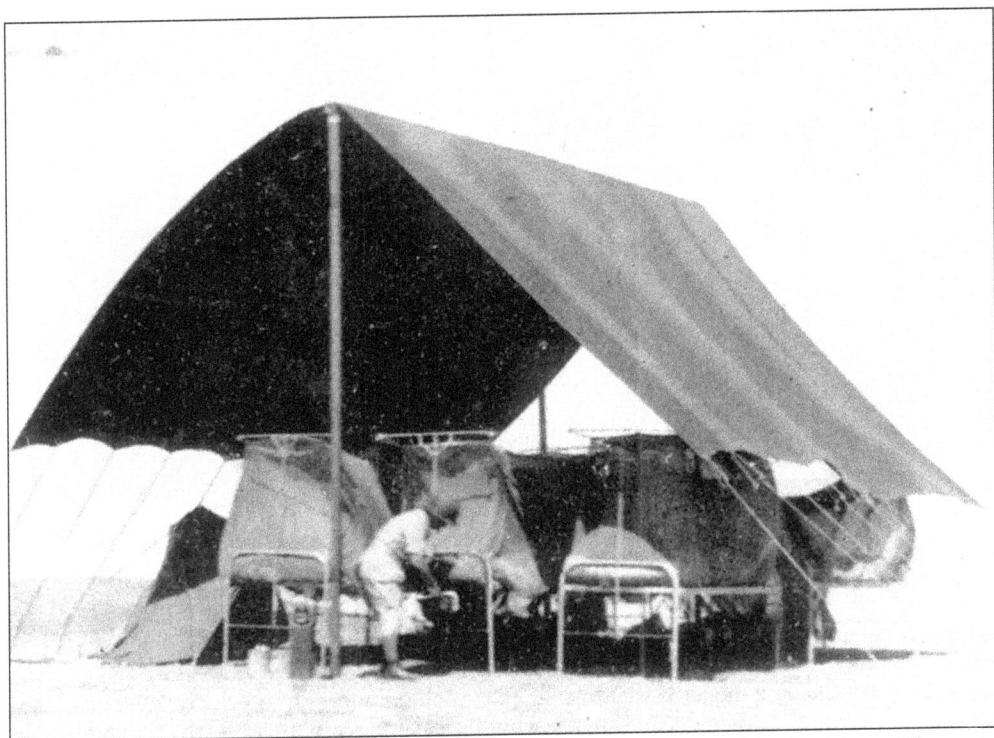

THE FIRST CASES AT BIZERTE. Nine months were spent in Bizerte, North Africa. There, in January and February 1944, sleet and hail blew down several ward tents, and patients were moved to less fragile structures. The 33rd General Hospital then served in Rome for four months and at Leghorn, Italy, for a year. Also of note, a team of four nurses was instituted to ensure accurate and prompt administration of the new drug penicillin.

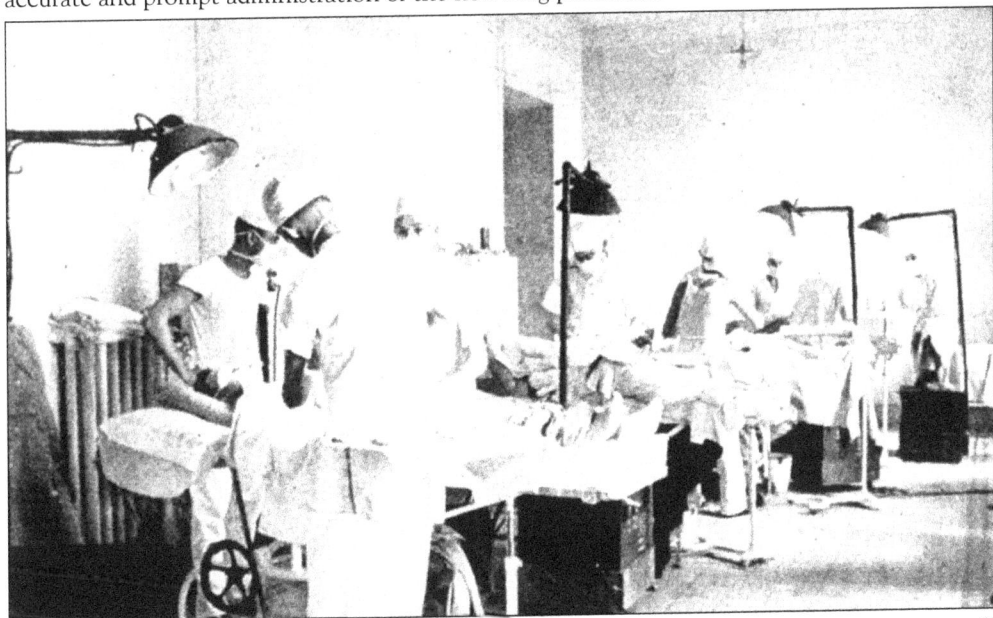

FOUR SURGERIES IN PROGRESS. When casualties came in droves, it was necessary to use all available space and staff to care for the emergency needs of the wounded.

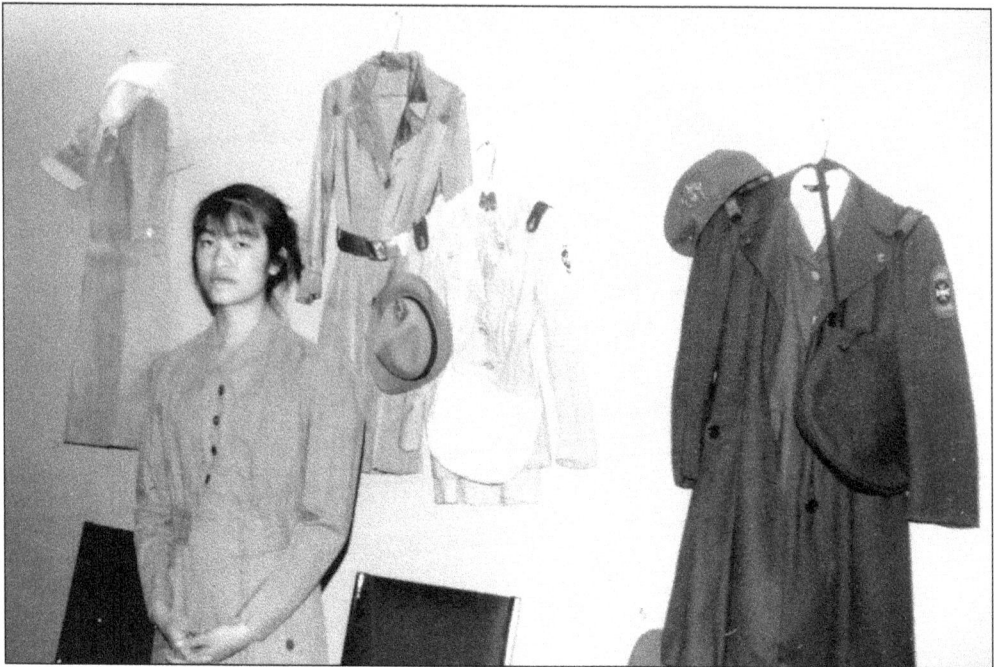

CADET UNIFORMS. The model is wearing the blue probie uniform from which students gained the name "blue birds." Also pictured are the gray clinical uniform with a cap, the cadet raincoat, a summer cadet outdoor uniform, and a winter cadet outdoor uniform, which were donated to the Alumni Association by members of the 1947 RSCSN Cadet Nurse Corps in affiliation with Albany Hospital and Albany Medical College. (Courtesy Christine Howanski Lansing, R.N., Class of 1947.)

THE FIRST UUSN CLASS MEMBERS WERE CADETS. Gertrude King, Class of Spring 1948, applied for the U.S. Cadet Nurse Corps (see page 56). In fact, all 34 members of the class were cadets. Because the war ended, these students did not receive the cadet uniform or cadet pin but did receive all the other benefits of free tuition and stipends.

Federal Security Agency
United States Public Health Service
for Meritorious Service

IN RECOGNITION OF THE WARTIME CONTRIBUTION OF

Dorothy Connors

AS INSTRUCTOR FOR MEMBERS OF THE U. S. CADET NURSE CORPS

This Nation will always be indebted to the Instructors in Schools of Nursing who prepared the largest classes of student nurses in history for military and essential civilian nursing.

As an Instructor your influence will be reflected in each of the young women to whom you have imparted your skill, knowledge, and wisdom. Through them you have cared for hundreds of patients. You have produced the graduate nurses of tomorrow who will be a vital factor in the public health of our country and of the world.

Thomas Parran
Surgeon General.

AN ACKNOWLEDGEMENT FROM THE SURGEON GENERAL. Dorothy Connors, R.N., Class of 1936, received a certificate signed by the surgeon general acknowledging her wartime contribution as an instructor for members of the U.S. Cadet Nurse Corps.

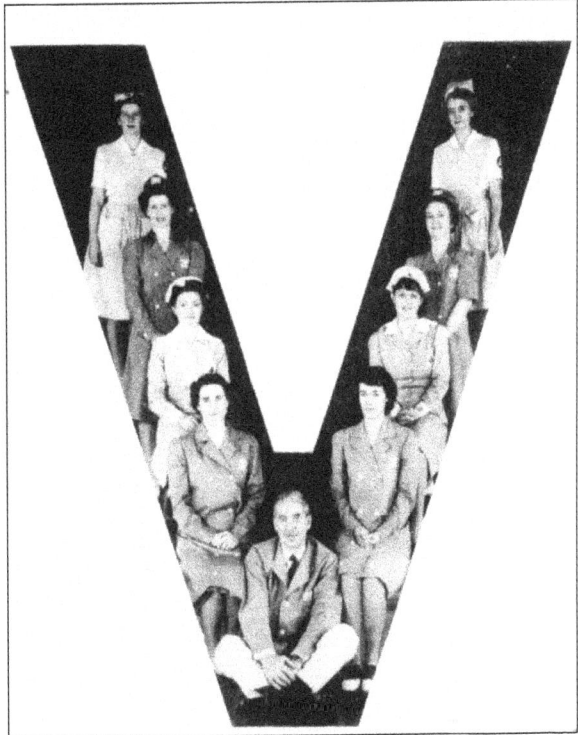

AN ALBANY HOSPITAL CHRISTMAS CARD TO VOLUNTEERS. The hospital sent this card to the volunteers in 1944 as a gesture of thanks for their many hours of service that eased the nursing shortage during World War II.

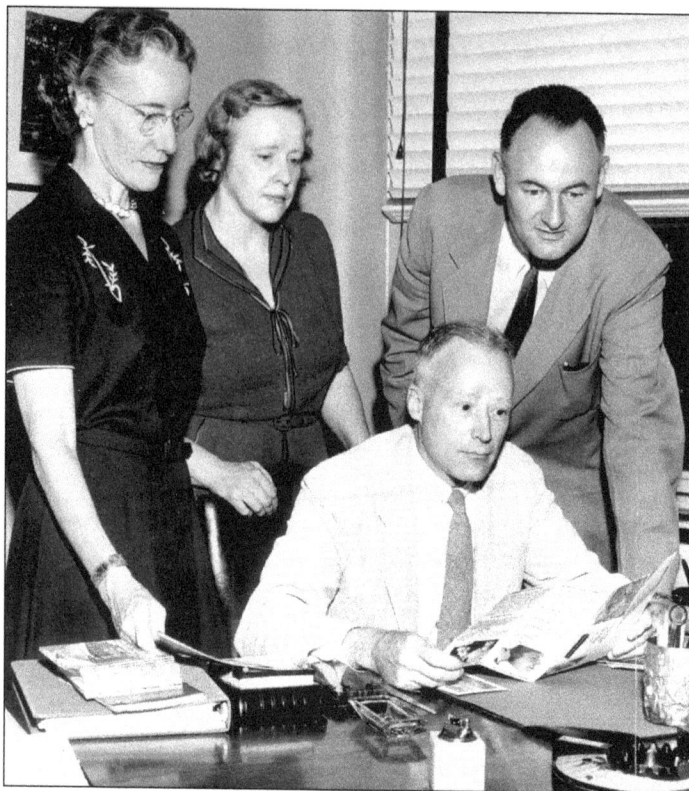

PLANS FOR UUSN. In 1954, Albany Hospital director Dr. Thomas Hale Jr., UUSN acting director Marion Wood, board of visitors member Mrs. Ten Eyck Powell, and Albany Medical College dean Dr. Harold Wiggers reviewed plans to reduce tuition, create a paid internship, and shorten the preclinical period for UUSN. Preliminary plans developed into the formation of AMCSN, a three-year diploma program under Albany Hospital's board of governors. (Courtesy *Knickerbocker News*.)

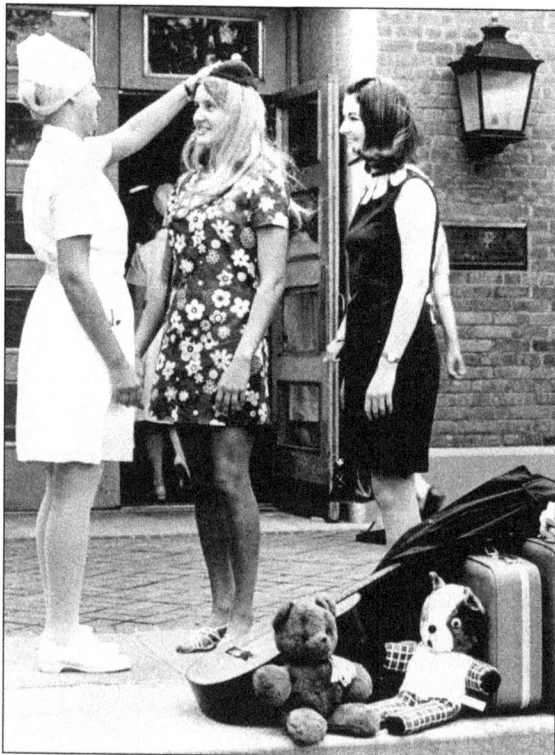

WELCOME NEW STUDENTS. A student in the big sister class greets a new student with an AMCSN beanie at the nurses' residence entrance. Students were welcomed to an atmosphere that stimulated intellectual curiosity and developed discipline essential to gaining and applying the knowledge and skills needed for nursing practice.

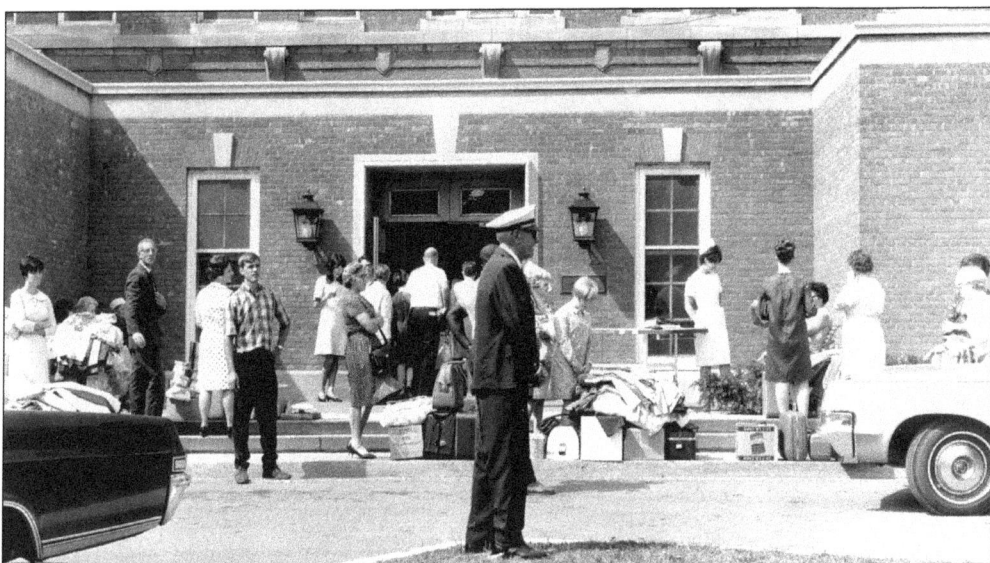

More New Class Arrivals. A circular drive led up to the residence doors, where anxious students were welcomed to the school. Years of personal treasures boxed to fit in one small room and all the hopes and dreams of students and parents were carried through this doorway. Here is where the journey began.

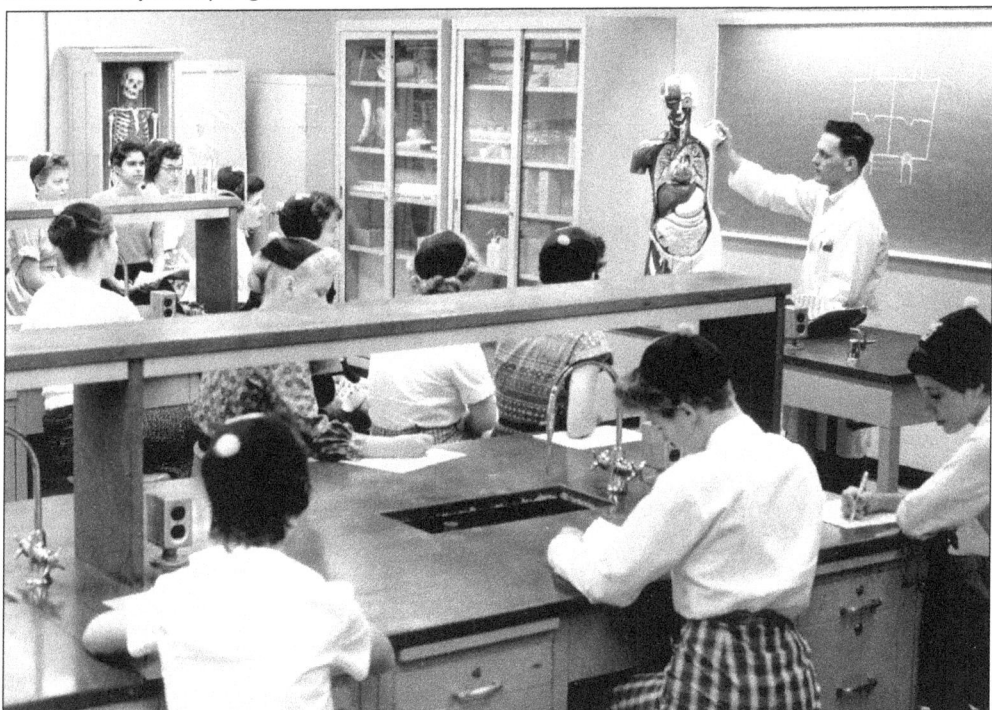

Classes Begin. Freshman students learned about all of the parts of the body, how they function, and what happens when they malfunction. Beanies still had to be worn at all times. The attire of the day was dresses or skirts and blouses. Many a student had slacks rolled up under their skirt until they were off campus and could shed the skirt, roll it up in a bag, and roll down the legs of the slacks.

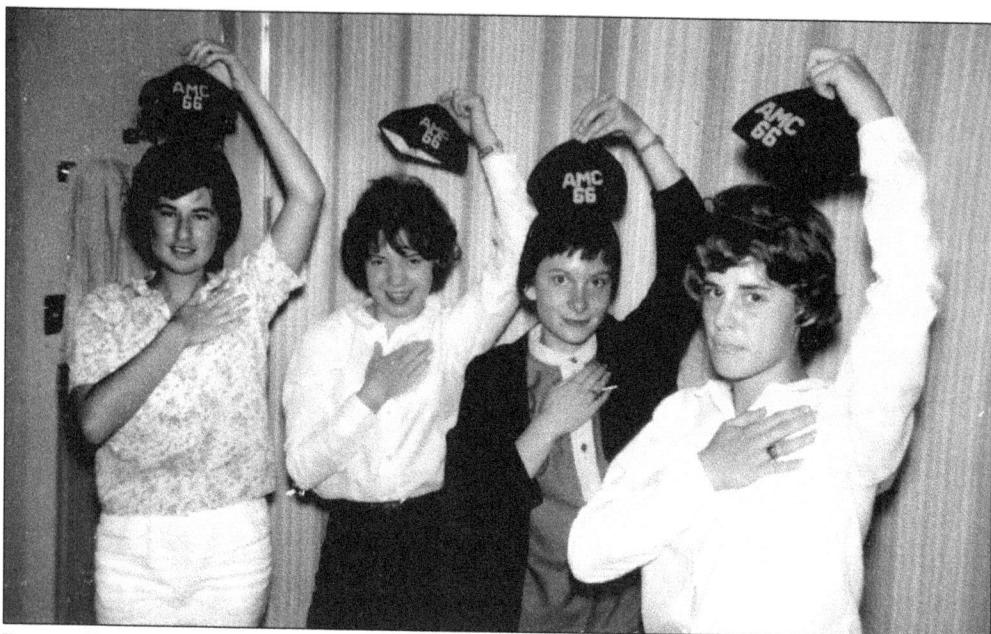

BEANIE BABIES OF THE 1960S. Freshmen from the Class of Fall 1966 tip their beanies to upper classmen and pledge to be true to their school. From left to right are Gail Groth, Bobbie Stenson, Christine Anderson, and Margaret Malec. (Courtesy Jane Saiff Williams, R.N., Class of Fall 1965.)

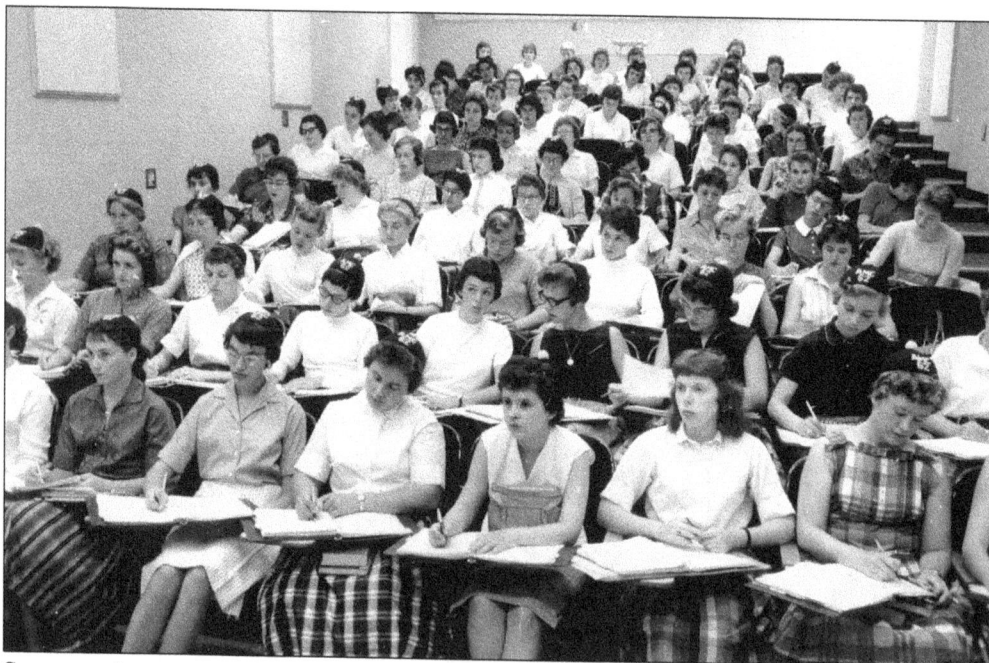

SAMPSON AUDITORIUM. Members of the Class of Fall 1962 take notes during a class lecture in Sampson Auditorium. Located in the nurses' residence, it had 105 seats and was named in memory of Dr. John Sampson (see pages 42 and 43).

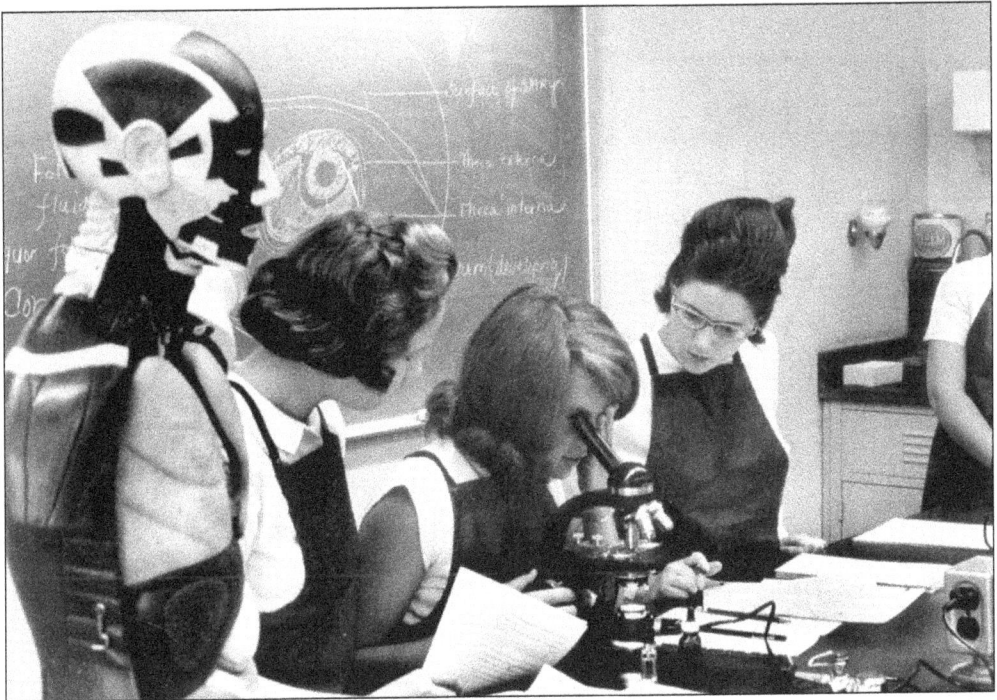

THE BASIC SCIENCES LABORATORY. Students use a microscope to study tissue samples of the ovary. The nursing program consisted of 146 weeks of education divided into three periods: freshman, clinical, and internship. Understanding organs' and systems' interdependence and interrelationship began with the molecular level and progressed to the body as a whole.

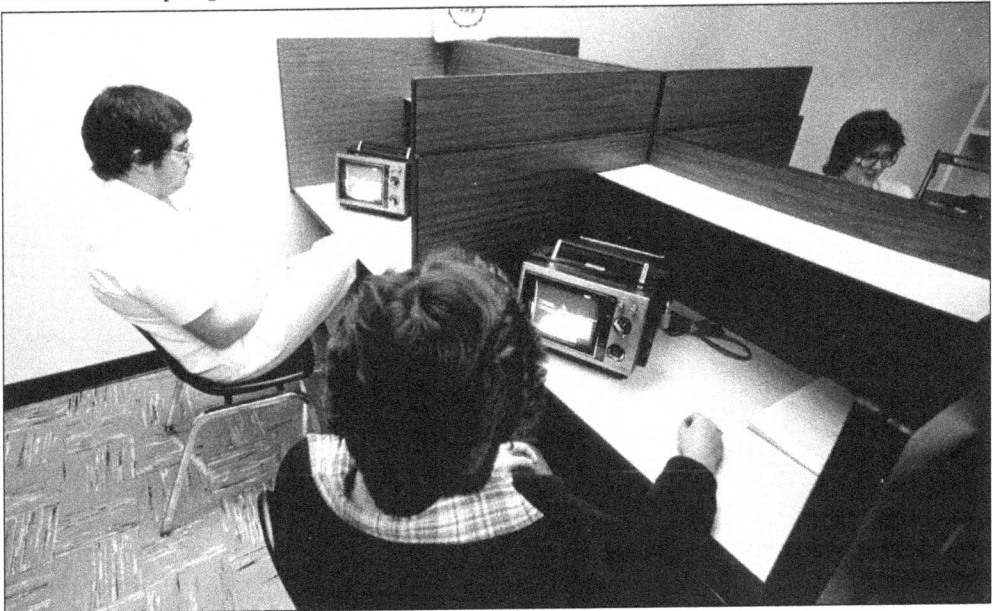

THE DONNA HAYES READING ROOM. This room was dedicated to Donna Hayes, a nursing student who died in 1971, four months before her graduation. A grant from the Helene Fuld Health Trust Fund gave the school audio-visual equipment for a self-tutoring program that was placed in the Donna Hayes Reading Room.

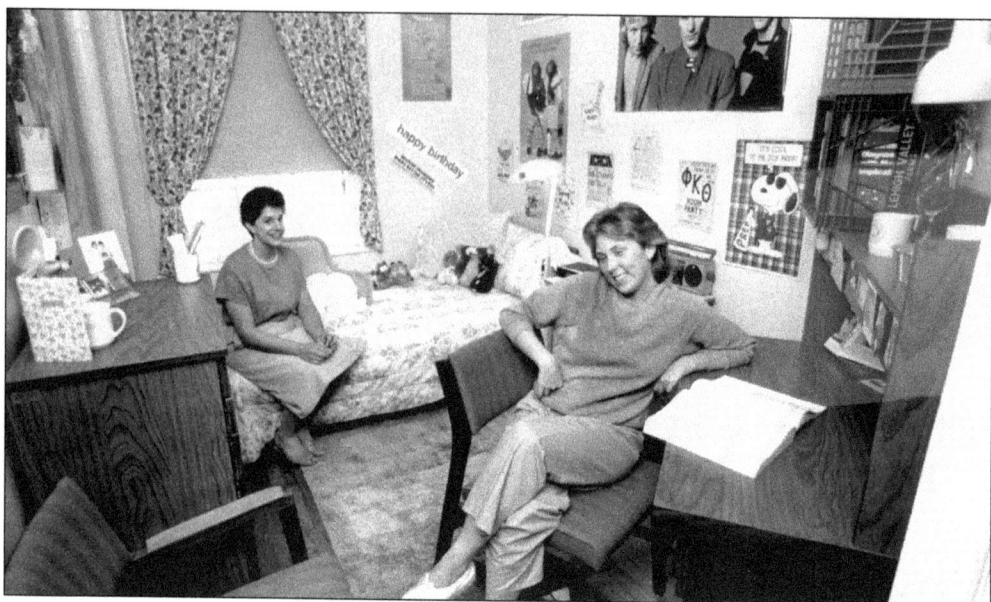

A RESIDENCE ROOM. A typical room in the residence was furnished with a bed, dresser, chair, and desk and was decorated to the student's taste. Visits to classmates' rooms were permitted, but no outside visitors were allowed except for family members at designated times. In the 1980s, students successfully petitioned for freedom from residence curfews and the liberalizing of visitation rules.

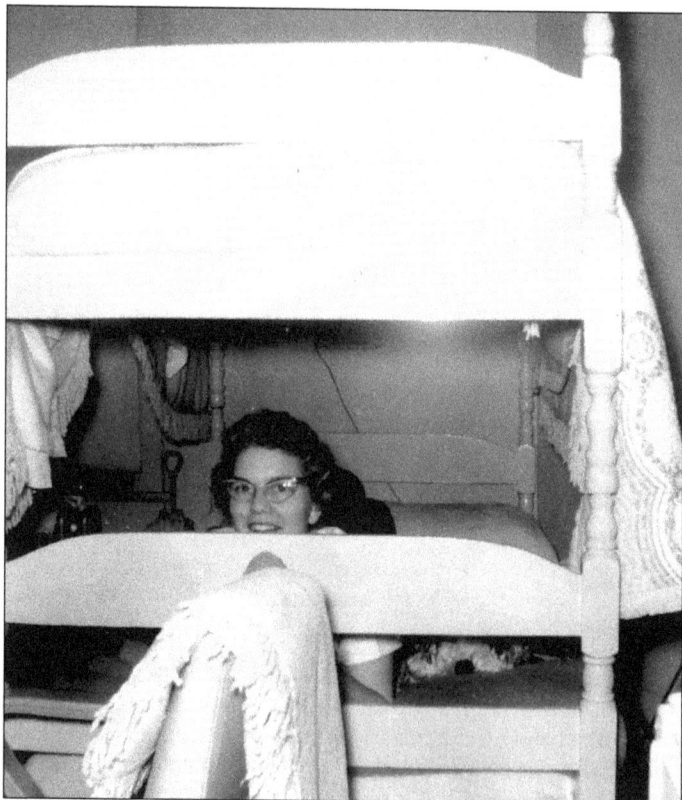

GETTING TO THE TOP. Because of increased enrollment, overcrowding in the residence sometimes required the use of bunk beds. Creativity was often needed when accessing dresser drawers and closets, as handles could become interlocked. There was one central phone on each floor. (Courtesy Marilyn Lasher Olmstead, R.N., Class of Fall 1963.)

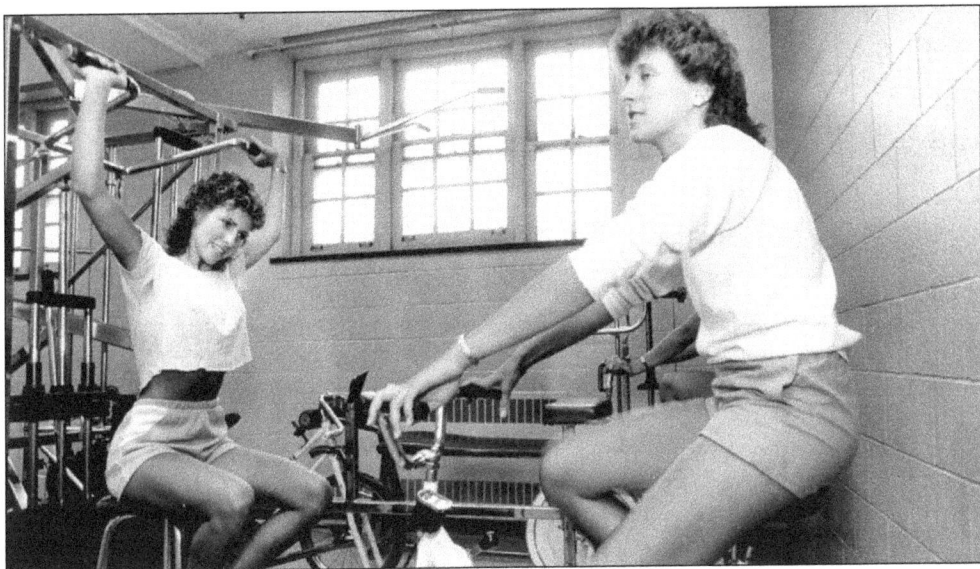

A UNIVERSAL GYM. In 1980, another grant from the Helene Fuld Health Trust Fund was used to renovate two bathrooms, redecorate the infirmary, purchase a large television, air-condition the student center, and obtain new classroom chairs. This fund, founded in memory of Helene Fuld, provided grants to schools of nursing for academic, dormitory, and recreational needs. An especially popular addition to AMCSN was a universal gym.

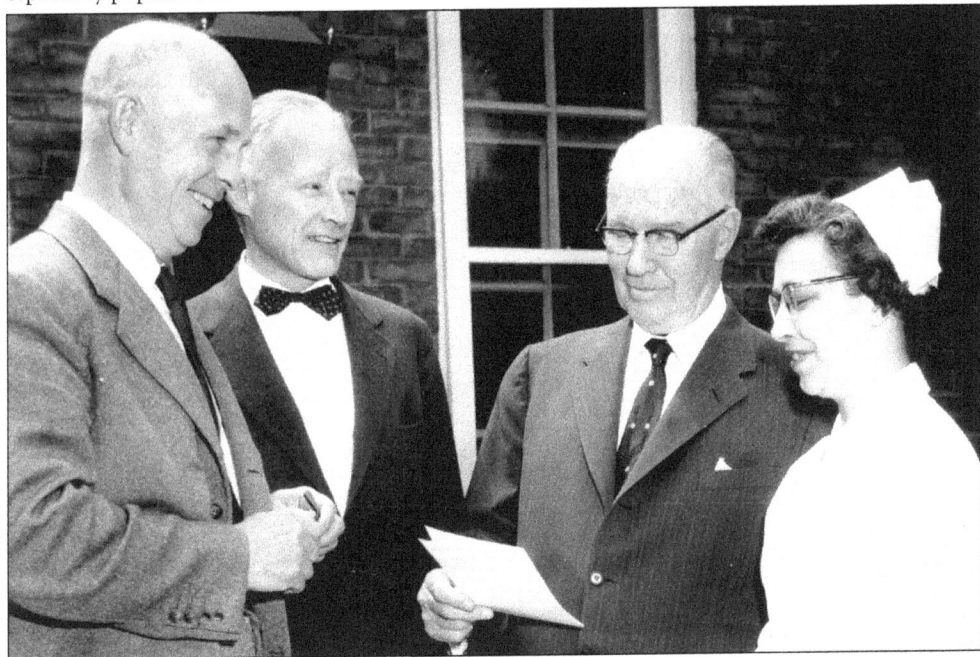

THE 1958 DEDICATION OF THE EDUCATIONAL UNIT AND MCDONALD LOUNGE. From left to right are board vice president Frank Wells McCabe, hospital director Dr. Thomas Hale Jr., board president Ralph Wagner, and director of AMCSN (1955–1972) Helen Flicker, R.N., participating in the dedication of the school's Sampson Auditorium (see pages 42 and 43) and McDonald Lounge. Frederick McDonald had the longest record of service of anyone then a member of Albany Hospital's board of governors.

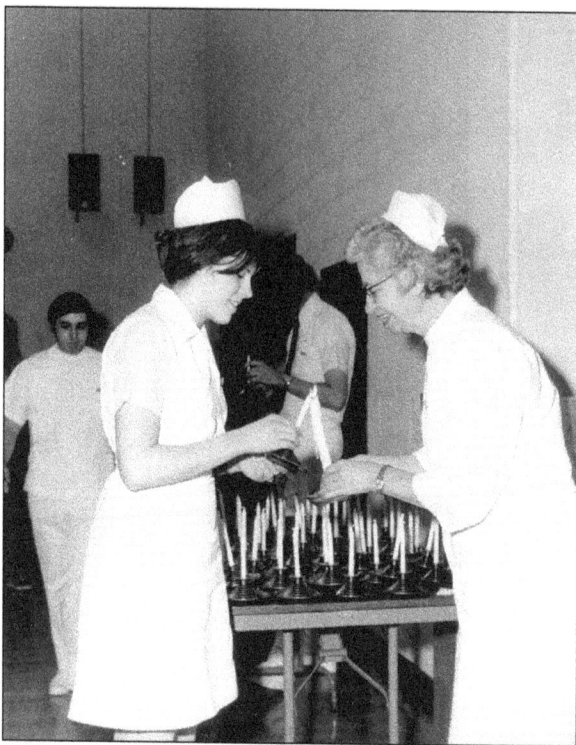

AMCSN CAPPING. The end of the probationary, or preclinical, period was celebrated by the capping ceremony. Verna Rolf, R.N., Class of 1937, the head of health service, holds the Nightingale candle lamp from which each student would light a candle. Rolf was a guiding force to all students until her retirement in 1984. Male students received a patch that they wore on their sleeve denoting that they were in their clinical term (see page 92).

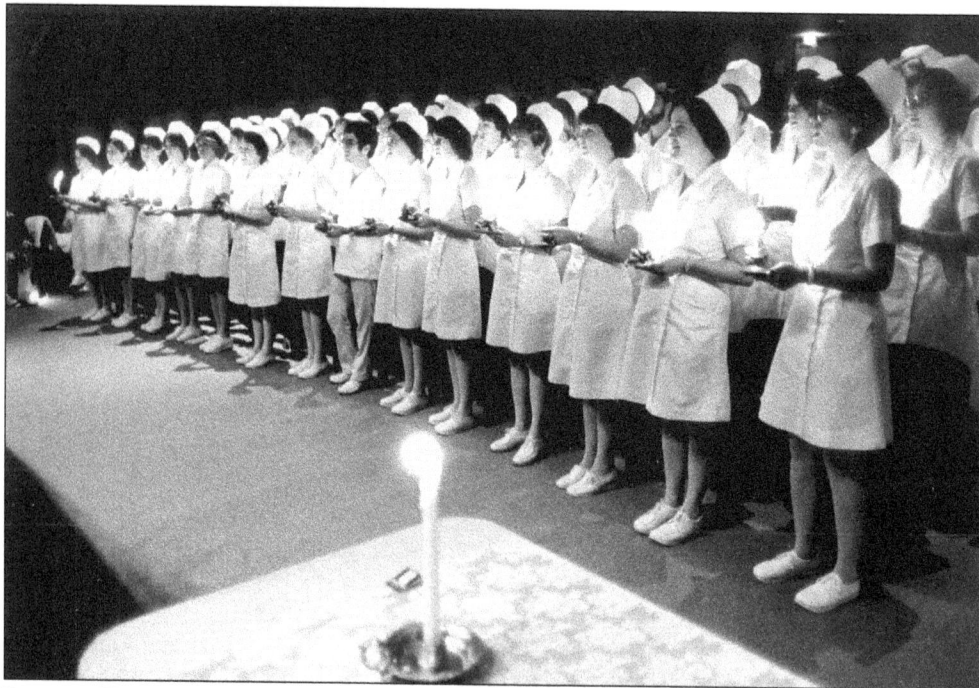

PASSING TRADITION AND PURPOSE TO THE NEXT GENERATION. At capping, each student lit a candle lamp, which symbolized the nursing profession. Traditionally, it has represented the day and night service and personal sacrifice reminiscent of Florence Nightingale, who used a lamp to light her way while making rounds among wounded soldiers.

ALBANY HOSPITAL BECOMES ALBANY MEDICAL CENTER HOSPITAL (AMCH). In 1967, Albany Hospital adopted the name Albany Medical Center Hospital. Accordingly, the Pillars Lobby entrance lettering changed from Albany Hospital to Albany Medical Center. AMCSN had been using the term "medical center" in its name since 1955.

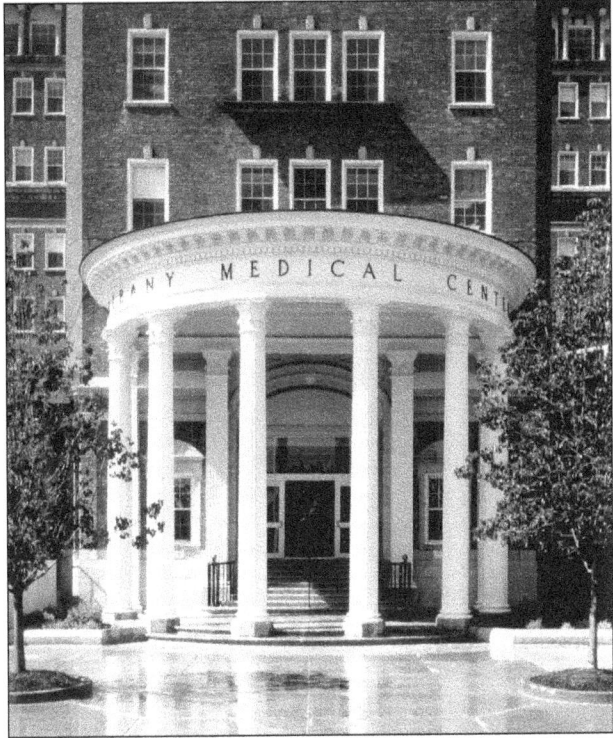

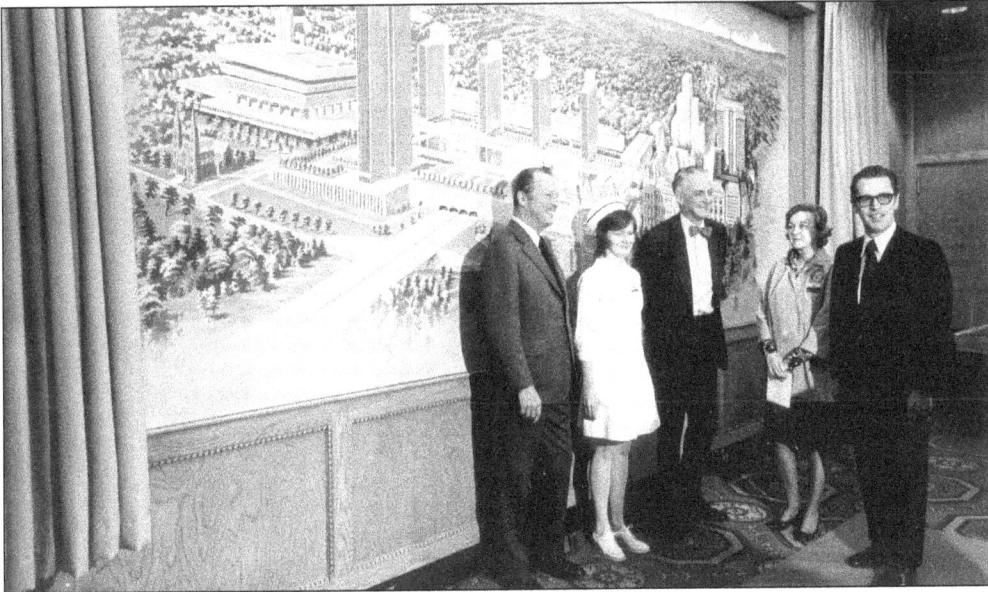

THE PILLARS LOBBY MURAL UNVEILING, MARCH 1975. Seen in this view are, from left to right, Maj. Gen. A. C. O'Hara, commissioner of the New York State Office of General Services; Mary Ann Lattanzio Patnode, R.N., Class of Fall 1968, representing nursing service; Dr. Thomas Hawkins, executive vice president of the hospital; Mrs. Frederick Elliott, president of hospital auxiliary; and George Pfaff, president of the hospital's board of governors. The mural of the Empire State Plaza in the Pillars Lobby is unveiled during dedication ceremonies. (Courtesy *Times Union*.)

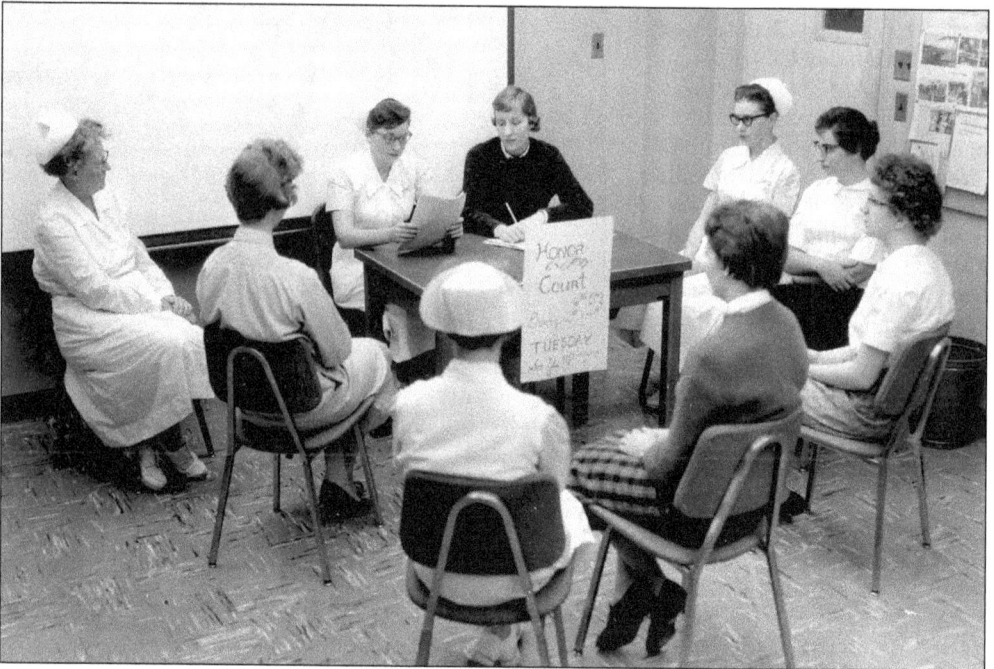

HONOR COURT. Honor court, sometimes called judiciary court, was composed of student representatives from each class and a faculty representative. Their duty was to uphold a democratic moral code that included areas of self government, professional and social life, and personal attitudes. Students who broke the rules came before the court to give their side of the story. A decision was made and, when necessary, demerits were given that resulted in loss of privileges.

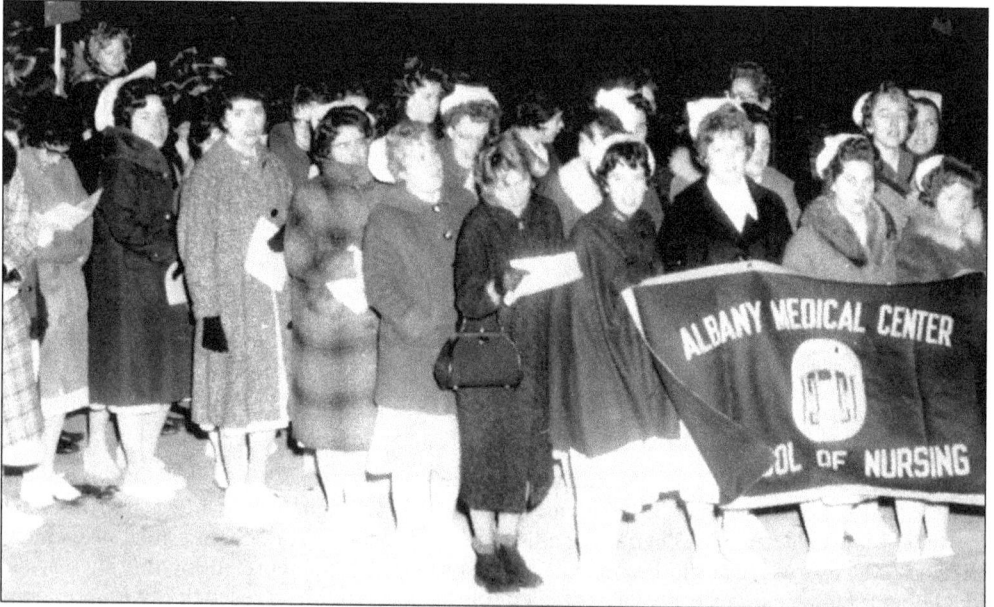

CHRISTMAS CAROLING. During the Christmas season, students would not only sing Christmas carols at AMCH but would also carry the school banner across New Scotland Avenue to sing at the Veterans Administration hospital.

A CARTOON OF AN AMCSN STUDENT. This pictorial of an AMCSN student appeared in the 1980 yearbook. Special equipment and multitasking were well known even then.

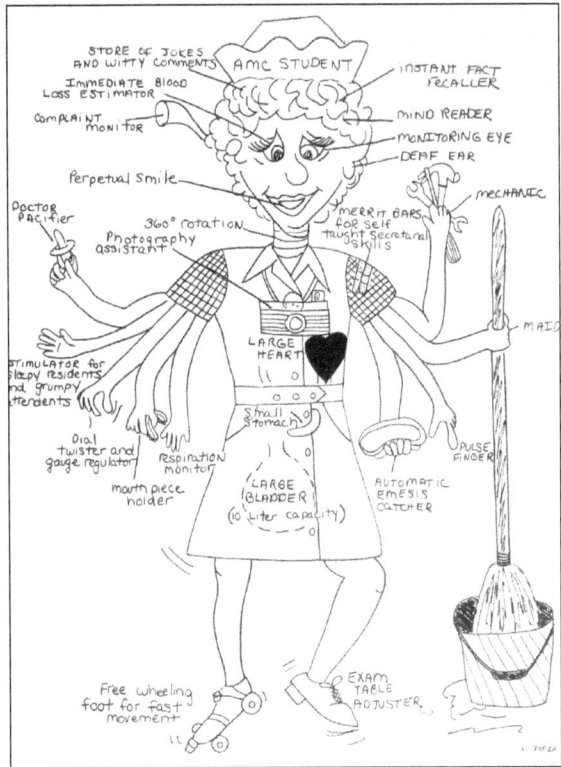

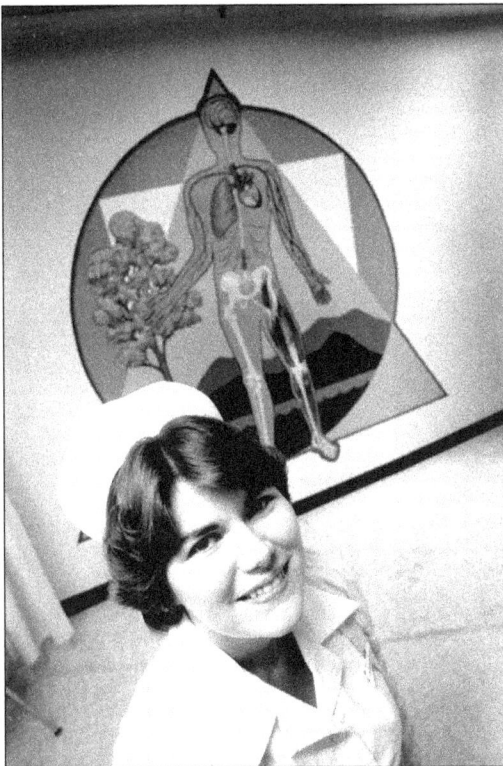

A MURAL IN THE STUDENT CENTER OF THE NURSES' RESIDENCE. Anna Conte, Class of Fall 1978, was a senior at AMCSN when she designed and painted this mural in the student center. It not only brightened the décor but expanded viewers' knowledge of anatomy as well.

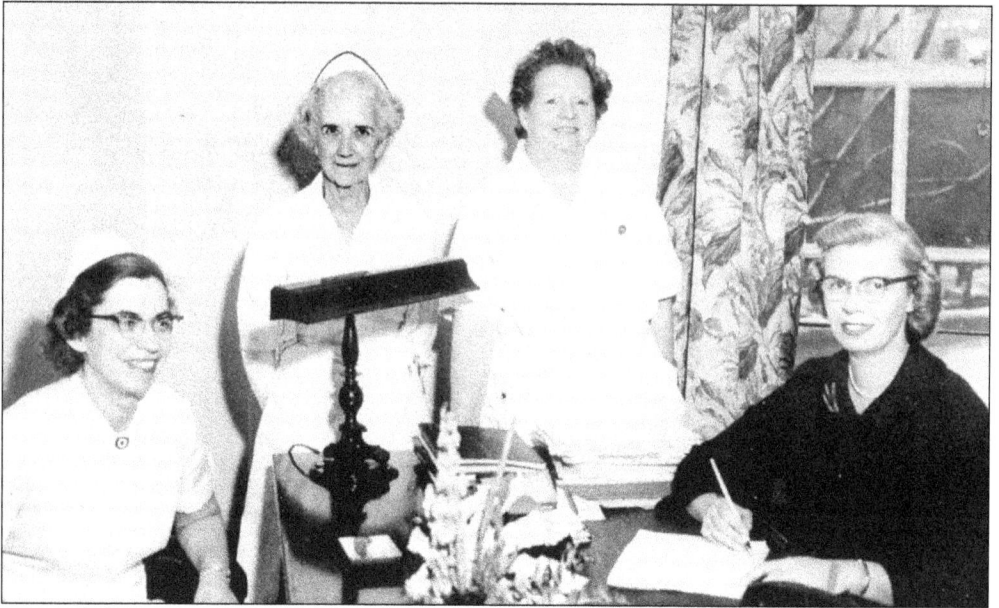

THE HEALTH SERVICE STAFF. These members of health service in 1959 are, from left to right, head nurse Verna Rolf, Mabel Keller, R.N.; Edna Paige, L.P.N.; and Marie Murray, M.D. They cared for the students as the students cared for others.

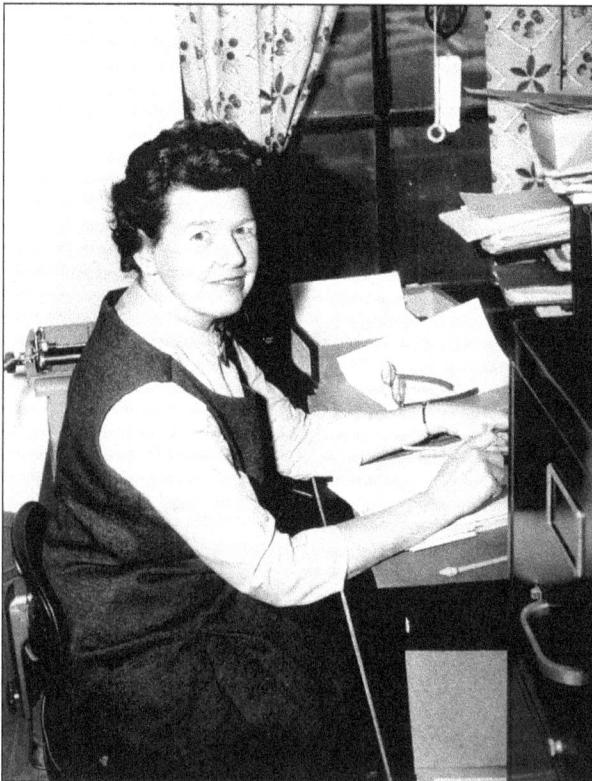

THE REGISTRAR. Evelyn Blackeby retired in 1976 after more than 33 years of faithful, productive service as registrar of UUSN and AMCSN. She always welcomed graduates by name when they returned for transcripts or a friendly visit. The accuracy of her records was legendary.

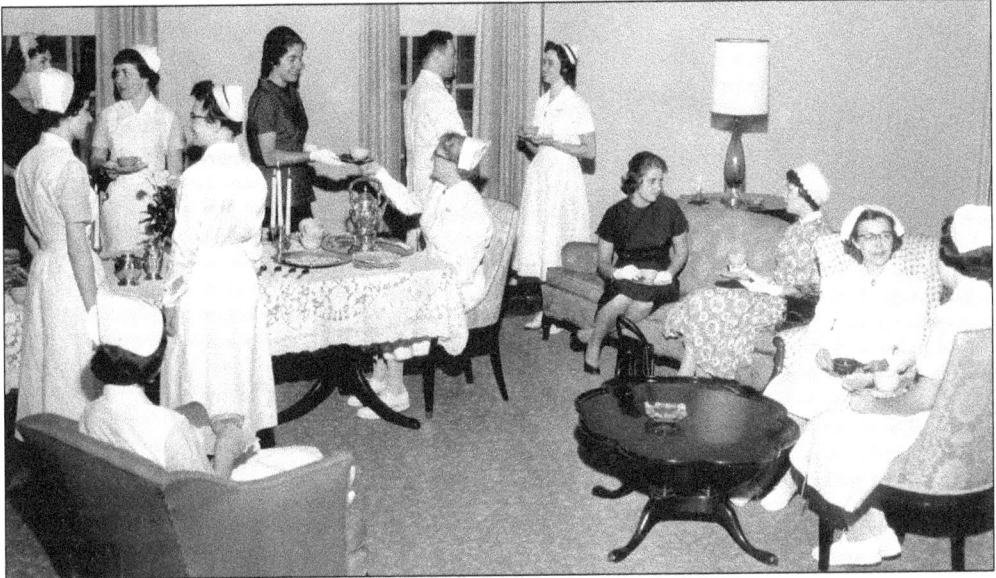

McDonald Lounge. In 1958, the new lounge in the nurses' residence was named McDonald Lounge in honor of Frederick McDonald, a member of the board of governors of Albany Hospital. It was used for capping and graduation receptions and formal social events. The dress of the day included a hat and gloves. Even as dress became more casual, the rule of "no jeans" remained a strict rule for McDonald Lounge attire.

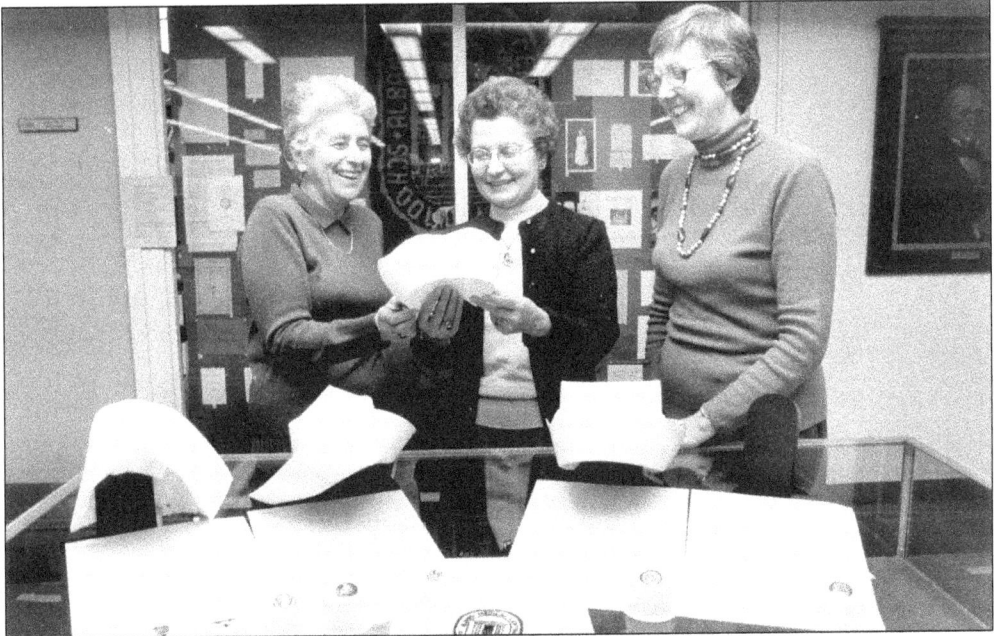

The Library Exhibit for the 25th Anniversary of AMCSN (1955–1980). Librarian Ursula Poland (left), AMCSN director Marie Treutler, R.N. (right), and assistant director Mary Gundrum French, R.N., Class of 1954, look over caps and pins from the schools of nursing. The caps, from left to right, are from AHTSN, RSCSN (worn by the U.S. Cadet Corps nurses), and UUSN. They are holding the AMCSN cap, which has four scallops representing the schools within the Alumni Association.

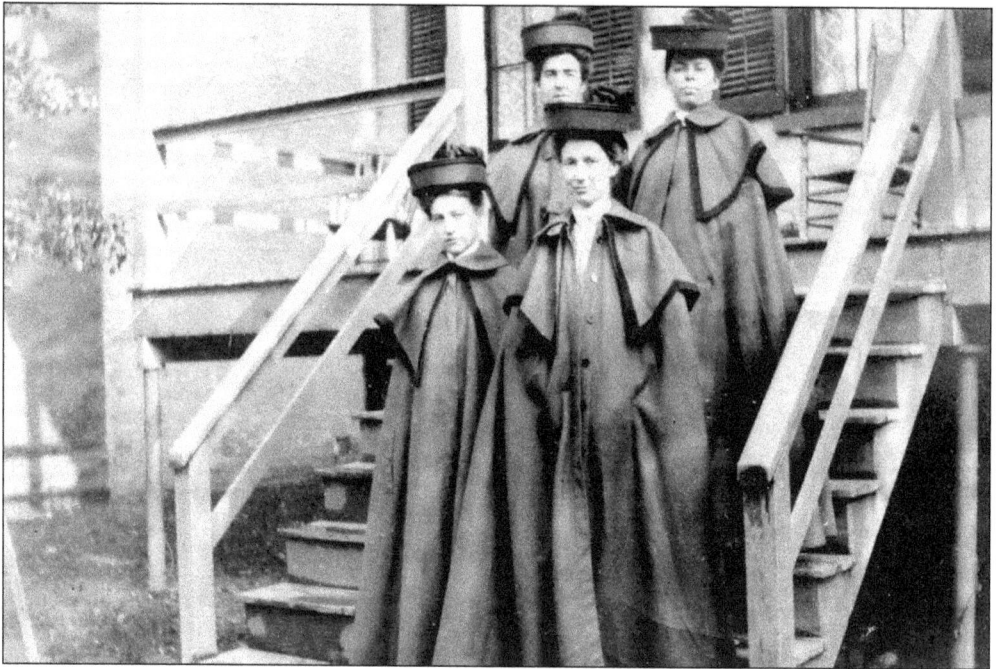

CERTIFIED NURSES. It would appear that outerwear and hats were part of the graduate certified nurses' uniform. This program was the forerunner of the practical nursing program.

The next term begins February 7, 1910

Circular of Information
of the
National Training School for
Certified Nurses
285 Lark Street, Albany, N. Y.

Designed to furnish a Six Month's Course of Scientific
Training for General Nursing

THIS SCHOOL IS ENDORSED BY THE MEDICAL SOCIETY OF THE STATE OF
NEW YORK, in the Report of its Committee on Training Schools, for year 1907 as
follows:—"There is a demand for nurses of more moderate education, who can give fairly
efficient service to those unable to pay the necessarily higher wages of the registered
nurse. The Albany school of nursing seems to be a reasonable attempt to furnish such
a class of women."

Correspondence should be addressed to
Dr. William O. Stillman, President.
287 State St., Albany, N. Y.

THE NATIONAL TRAINING SCHOOL FOR CERTIFIED NURSES 1907 CIRCULAR. A six-month course was designed to provide training for those wanting to gain nursing skills but unable to complete the three-year nursing program. These certified nurses provided care for those not requiring the services of a registered nurse.

No. 285 LARK STREET. This building was home for practical nursing students from 1905 until 1959, when it moved to a new hospital-owned building on Myrtle Avenue. Four months were spent at Glens Falls Hospital for medical, surgical, obstetric, and pediatric nursing and diet therapy.

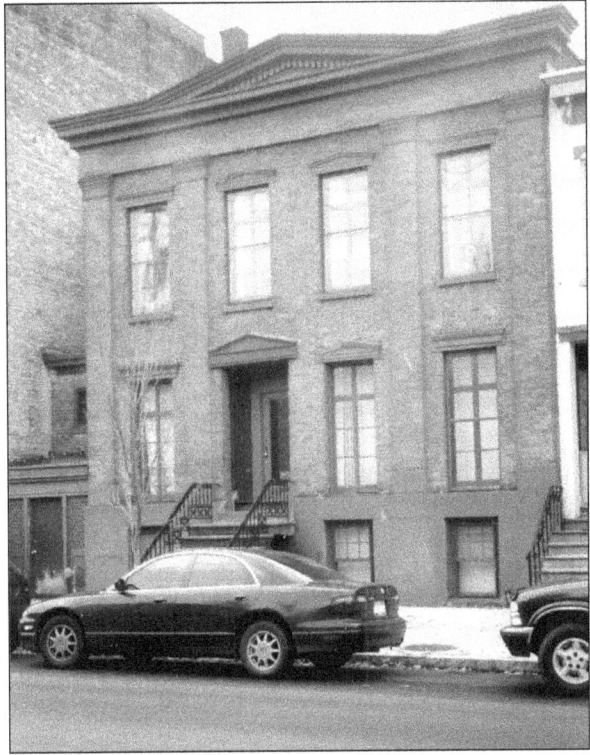

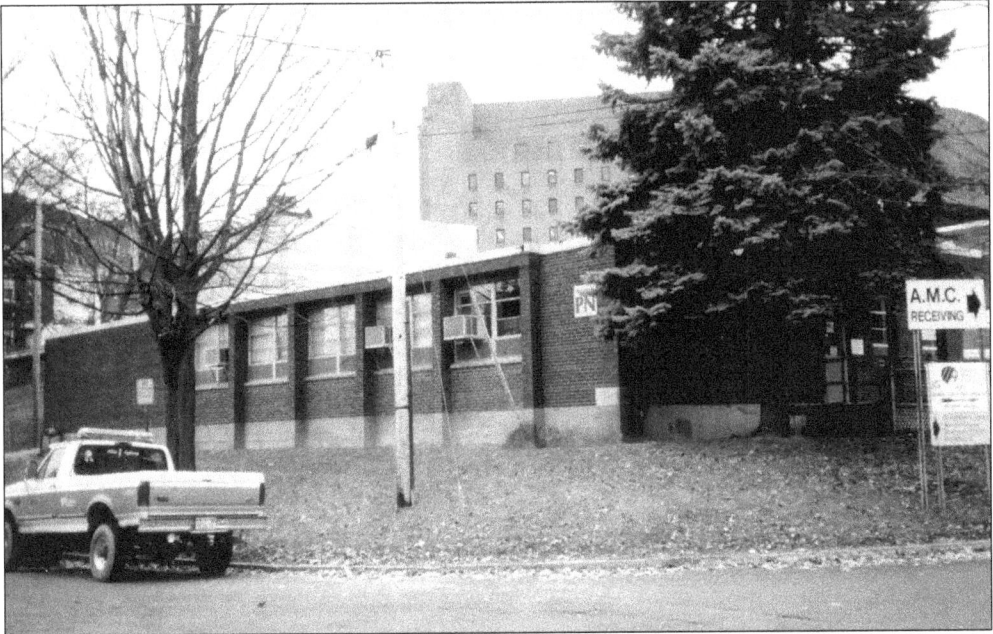

No. 470 MYRTLE AVENUE. In 1959, the name of the Albany Training School for Practical Nurses was changed to the Albany School of Practical Nursing. It was affiliated with Albany Hospital and located in the building at 470 Myrtle Avenue. The program was one year in length and cost $120 plus uniforms, books, and the students' own living arrangements. High school graduates were preferred, and the high school equivalency test was acceptable.

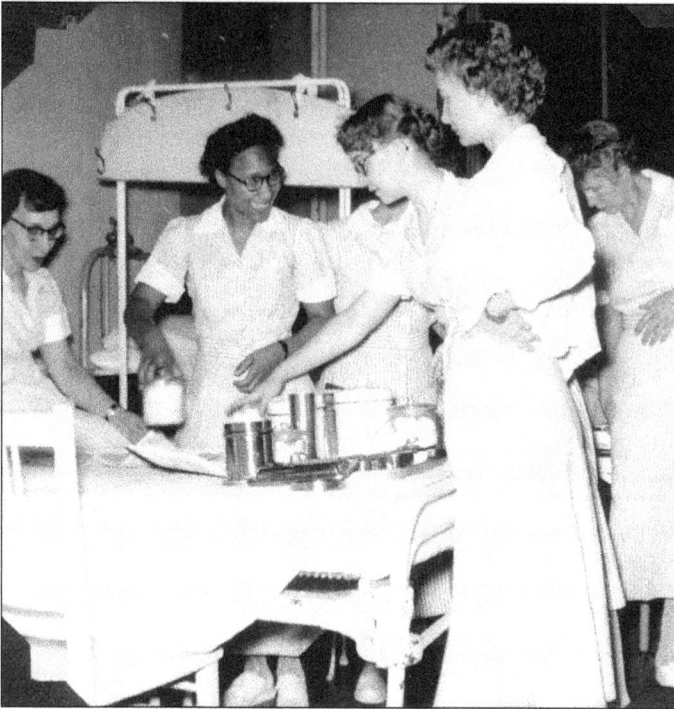

THE ALBANY SCHOOL OF PRACTICAL NURSING, c. 1957. From left to right, practical nurse students Charlotte Stockwell, Princess Flood, Dawn Thomas, and Marion Young are shown setting up a dressing change tray under the watchful eye of their instructor. Graduates took the New York State licensing exam to become licensed practical nurses (L.P.N.). Working under the supervision of a registered professional nurse or physician, they have contributed greatly to patient care. (Courtesy Janet Gilbert Gardner, R.N., Class of 1954.)

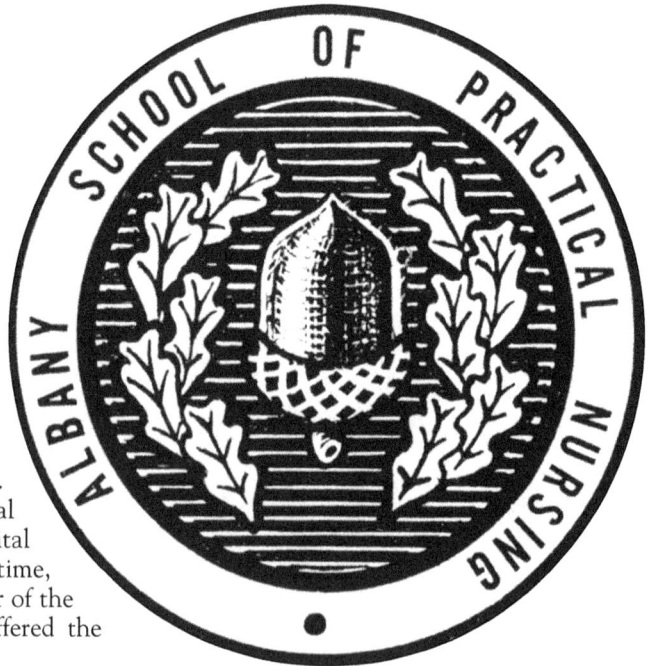

THE ALBANY SCHOOL OF PRACTICAL NURSING PIN. The distinctive pin depicts the potential strength of the acorn as it matures into a sturdy oak. The Albany School of Practical Nursing at Albany Hospital continued until 1974. At that time, the Albany Occupational Center of the Albany City School District offered the course for practical nursing.

A MOST IMPORTANT SKILL LEARNED.
Caring for a patient requires good listening and hearing skills to understand what the body, mind, and spirit of the patient are trying to tell you. Understanding their life, in the context they live it, is vital to developing a care plan that will meet their needs. This is the true art of nursing.

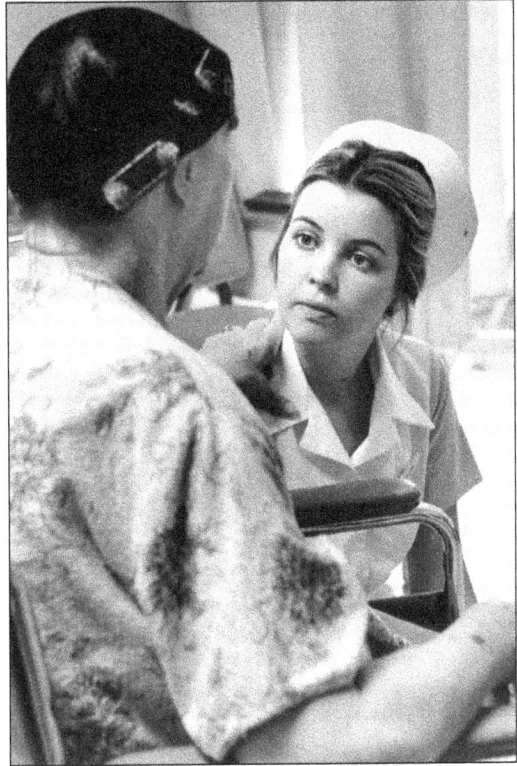

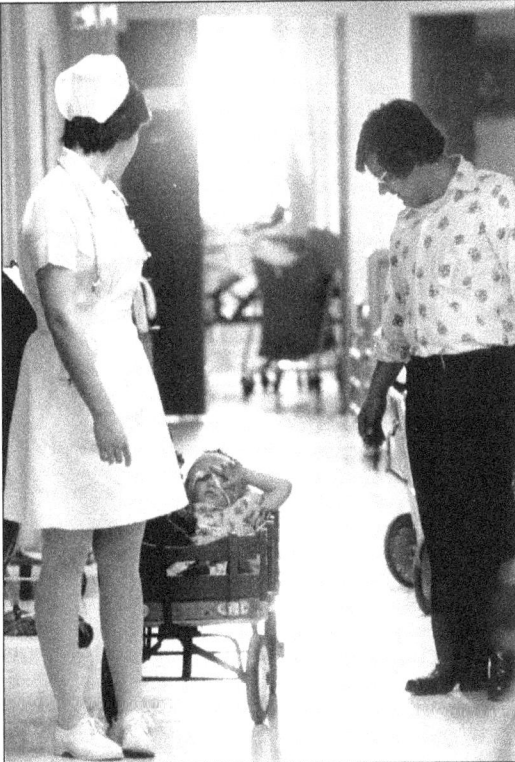

WHY NOT HAVE WAGONS IN A HOSPITAL? Paula Zenzen, Class of Spring 1966, gives this pediatric patient a ride in a wagon as Dad looks on approvingly. This method of transportation has been very popular over the years and gives the patients a feeling of home.

91

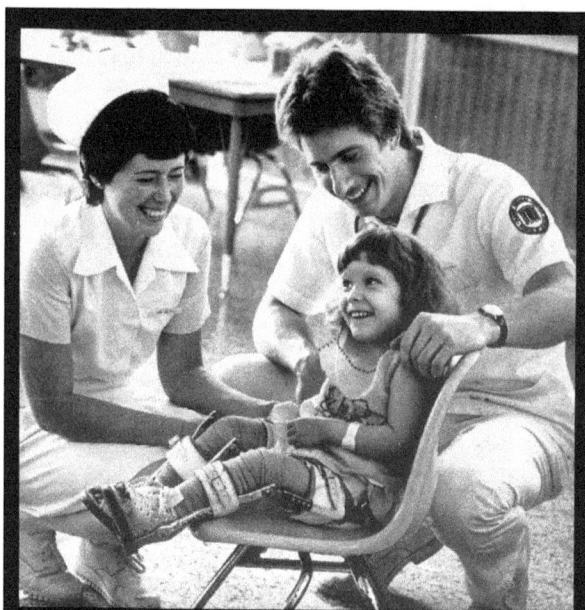

AN AMCSN CATALOG. AMCSN started in March 1955 with an enrollment of 10 students. Class members Christine Bianchi Leis and Dorothea Behm Bisceglia wrote the alma mater in Gregorian chant, and Judy Carpenter designed the school emblem and seal. Tuition for three years was $425 and included free uniforms, room and board, and a monthly stipend during the senior internship. At one point, AMCSN was the largest diploma school in New York State.

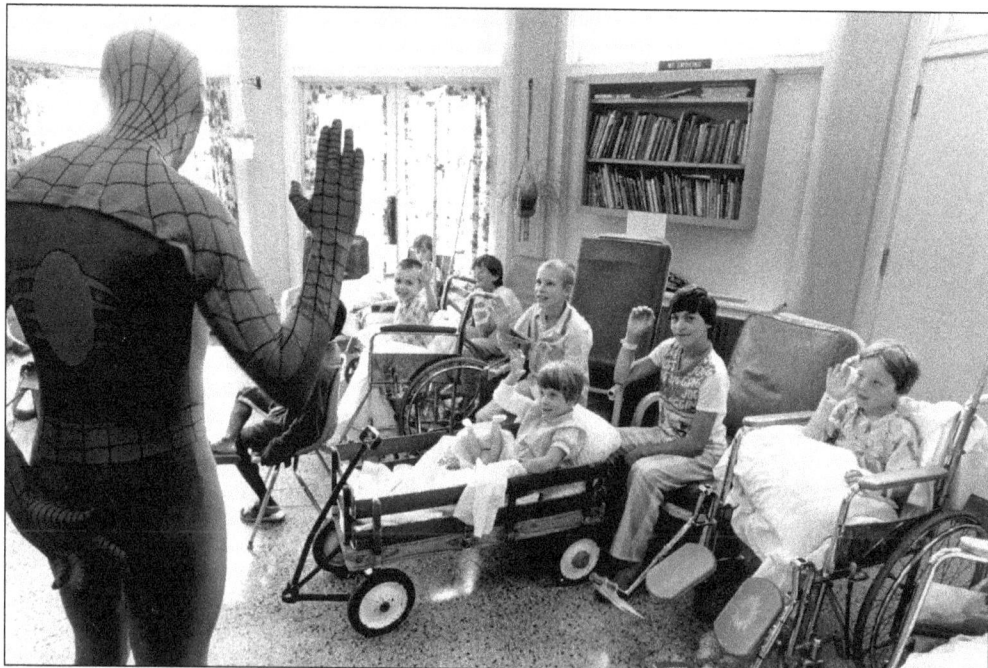

SPIDERMAN. The pediatric unit enjoys a visit from the well-known action figure Spiderman. Frequent visits from cartoon characters, sports figures, and holiday representatives all helped to provide welcome relief from the hard-to-bear part of care.

UP ON THE ROOF. Patients and staff enjoyed fresh air and sunshine on their rooftop getaway right off the playroom of the pediatric unit on Main 6.

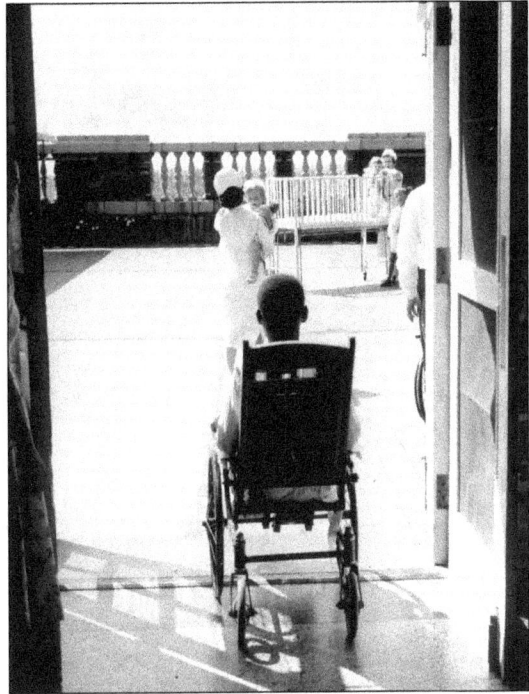

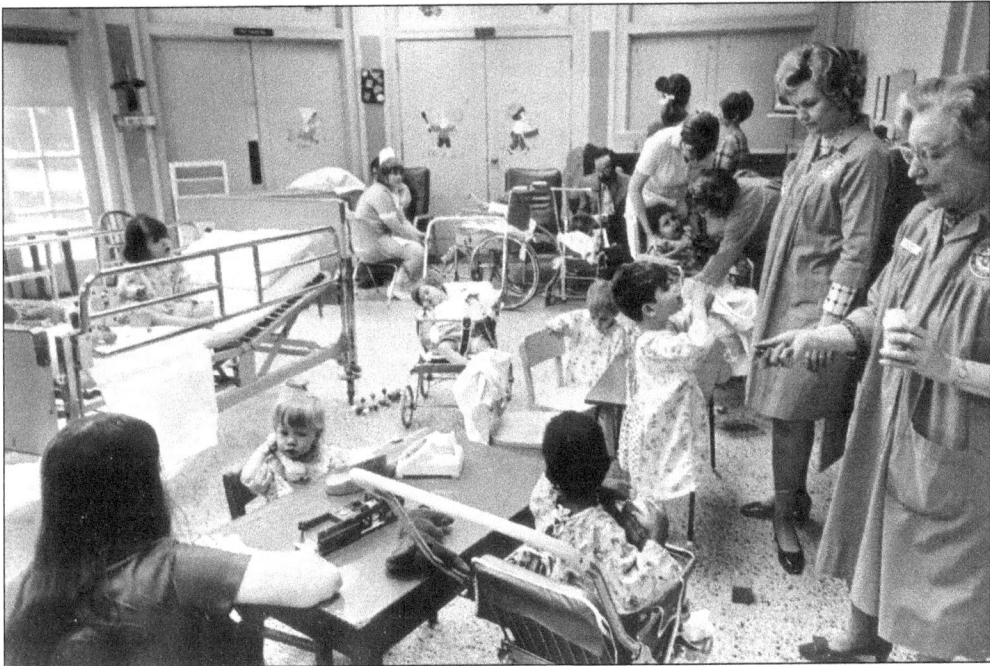

THE MEDICAL CENTER AUXILIARY. Volunteers, the ladies in cherry-red or men in the blue smocks, have provided tremendous assistance to staff, families, and children throughout the years. They provide a lap to sit on, hugs and laughs, or carriage and wheelchair rides. They operate the thrift shop, patient library, and pediatric playroom. Beginning in 1969, the auxiliary gave a full-tuition scholarship to a deserving AMCSN student. From 1972 until the school closed, they increased their donation to include two full-tuition scholarships.

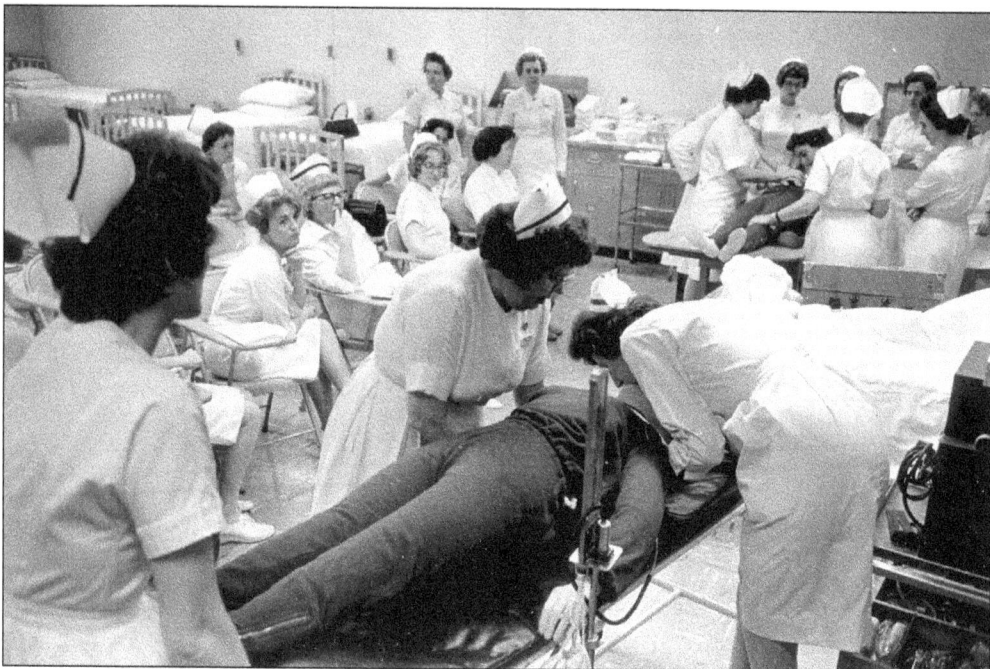

CONTINUING EDUCATION. Learning and maintenance of skills did not stop at graduation. A multitude of programs such as the cardiopulmonary resuscitation class (CPR) shown here were regularly offered to nursing staff. Rapid scientific development continually spurs the desire of nurses to excel in the application of new knowledge to practice.

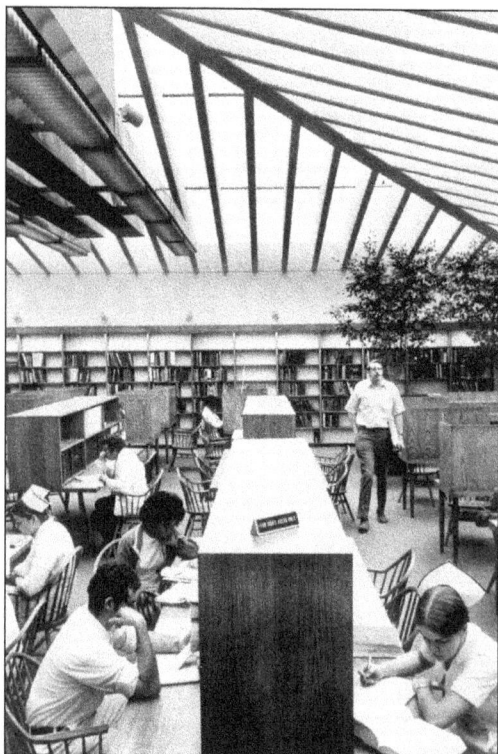

THE SCHAFFER LIBRARY OF HEALTH SCIENCES. In 1972, the library moved to the west side of the Albany Medical Center complex. Students could use rooms with slides, tapes, films, computers, and other communication media to pursue their studies. The large section of nursing volumes and periodicals is aided by an AMC Schools of Nursing Alumni Association annual fund drive.

FLUID BALANCE. An instructor explains physiological alterations in fluid and electrolyte balance in the administration of intravenous therapy. In 1973, an affiliation with the Junior College of Albany for six college courses was begun for a total of 21 college credits. In 1983, AMCSN contracted with the College of St. Rose for five three-credit courses.

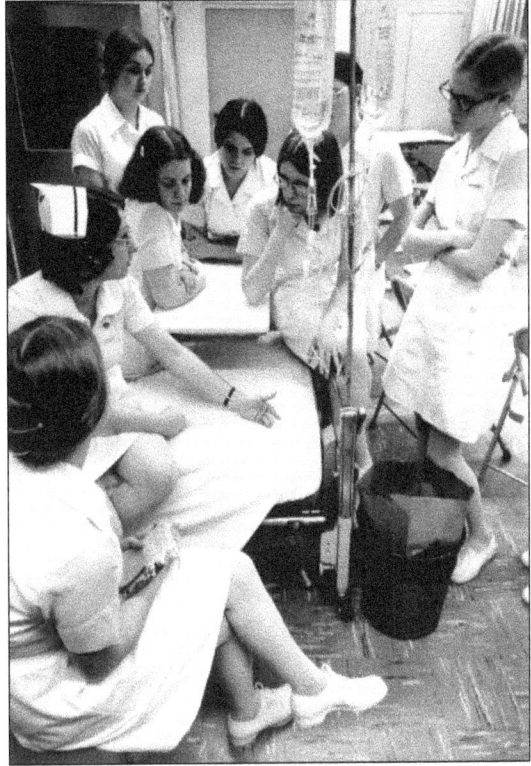

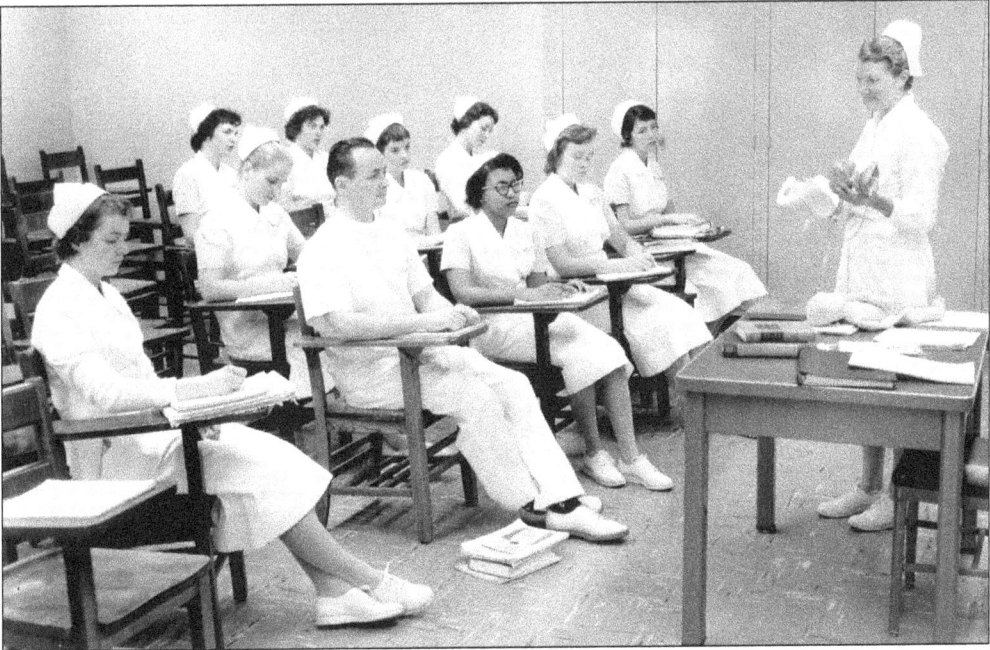

MATERNITY. Kathryn Burtt Golding, R.N., Class of 1936, taught obstetrical nursing to second-year students. Students looked forward to this class as a change from the focus on disease processes to that of the miracle of life and maintaining wellness in the family's natural life cycle. Tony Schmidt, shown here, was the first AMCSN male nursing student. He graduated in 1961.

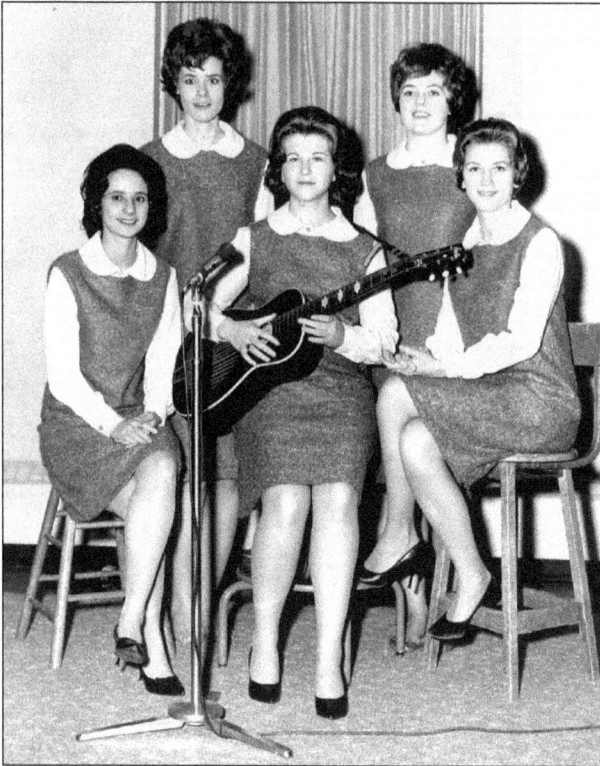

THE TRADEWINDS. From left to right, Reba Rettig, Sharon DeLisio, Patricia Potter, Linda McGuire, and Helen Price, members of the Class of Spring 1964, formed the Tradewinds, a singing group that made its debut at an AMCSN talent show. The Tradewinds' arrangements were patterned after those of Peter, Paul, and Mary and Harry Belafonte. Dinner performances, recordings, and radio appearances followed.

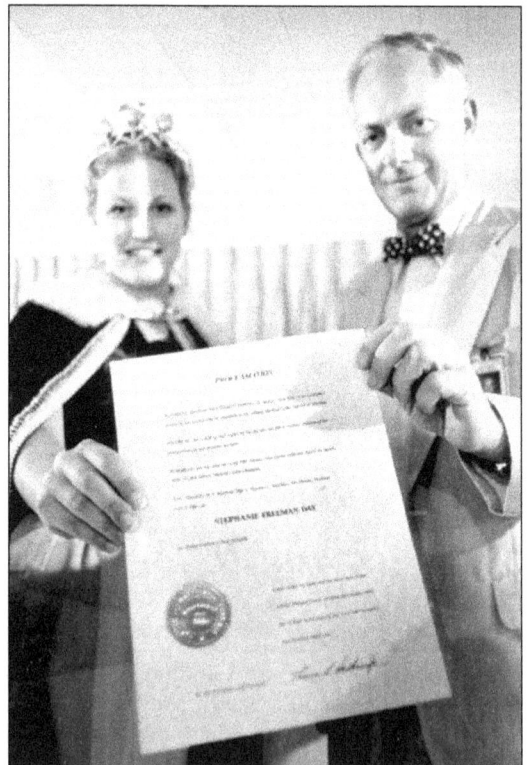

THE 1961 TULIP QUEEN. Seen here are Stephanie Freeman, Class of Fall 1962, and Dr. Thomas Hawkins Jr., director of AMCH. Freeman is wearing her crown and cape as she and Hawkins display the proclamation announcing June 3, 1961, as Stephanie Freeman Day at AMCH. The Tulip Festival continues to be held every spring in Albany to celebrate the city's Dutch heritage. Another celebration tradition that continues to this day is the scrubbing of State Street by industrious ladies in Dutch costume.

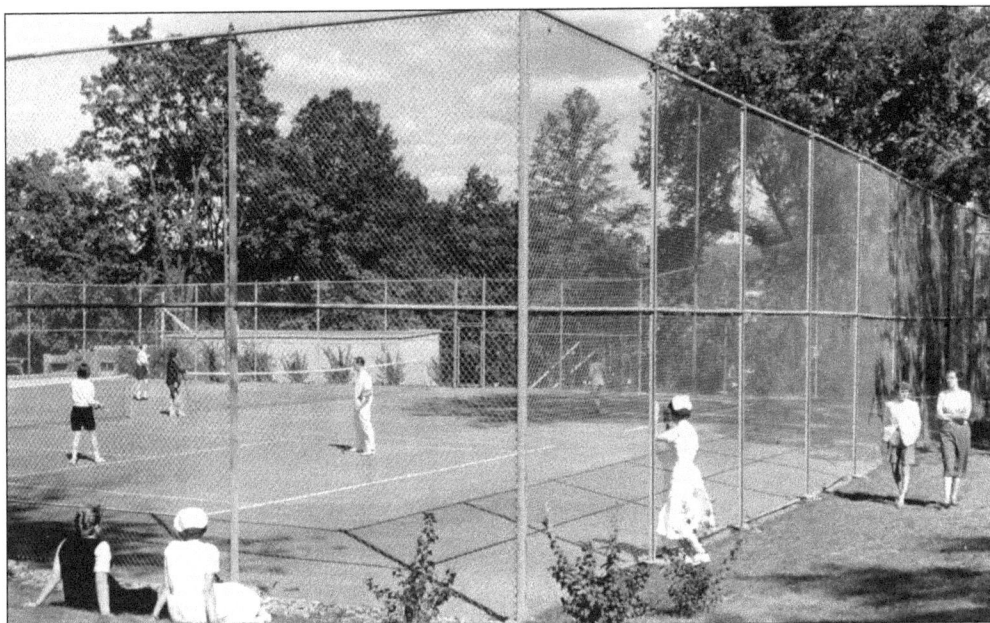

TENNIS, ANYONE? Fun and games were an important part of team building and camaraderie as well as relaxation. The sports committee maintained a room for sports equipment and also promoted swimming, basketball, baseball, horseback riding, bowling, fencing, and bicycling. The two tennis courts were donated by the Albany Hospital Women's Auxiliary in 1959.

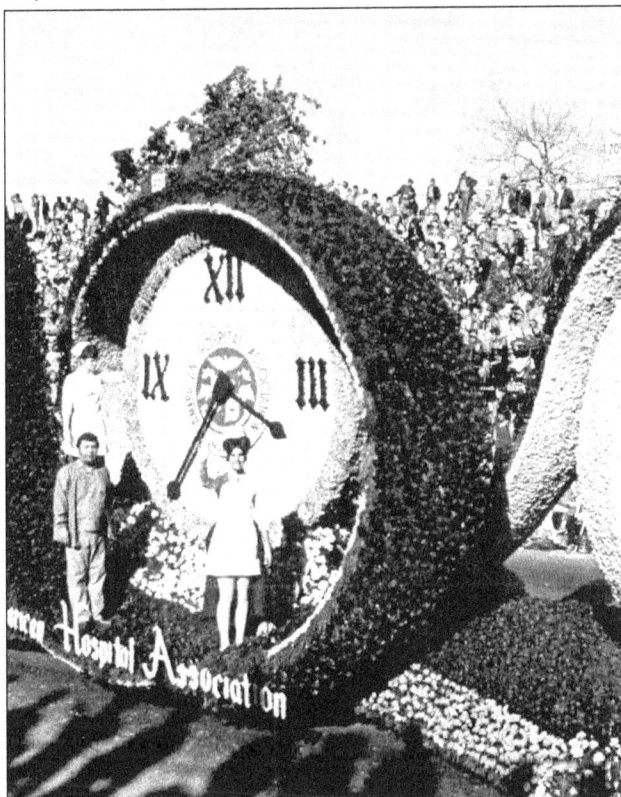

THE TOURNAMENT OF ROSES PARADE. Marie Treutler, R.N., director of AMCSN, selected the winning ticket for the school to be represented on the American Hospital Association float in the 1972 Tournament of Roses parade. Sharon Buehler, R.N., Class of Fall 1966, who was then the Alumni Association president, was chosen to ride on the float, which had the theme of round-the-clock care. Buehler, facing the camera, smiles in spite of her allergy to flowers. (Courtesy the American Hospital Association.)

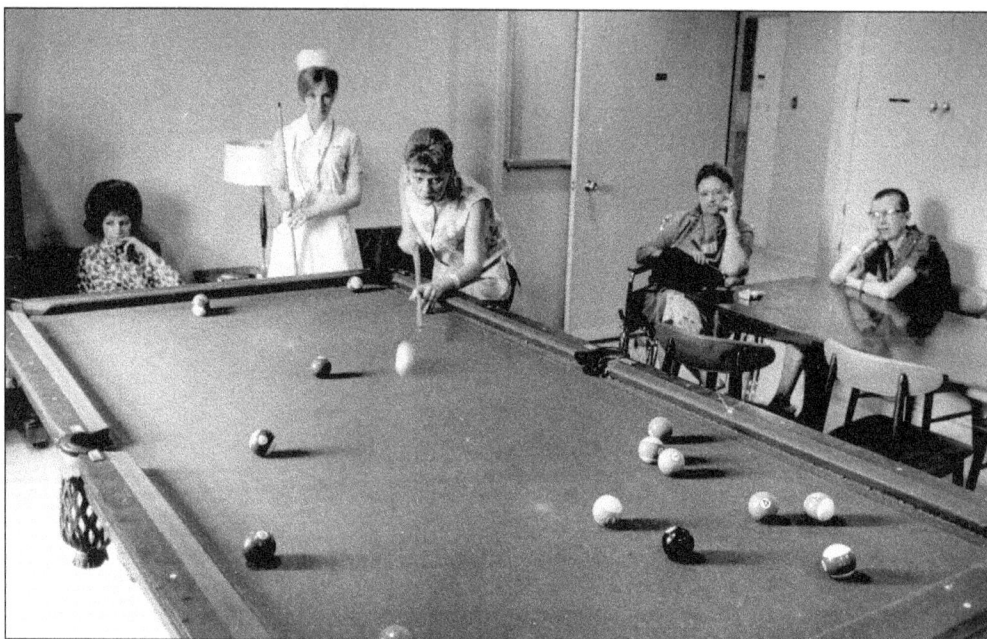

MOSHER MEMORIAL UPDATE. From the time the psychiatric units opened in 1902 until 1957, both the male and female units were locked. They then became coed and renamed as units F1 and F2, with F1 being the locked unit and F2 the open one. The pool table had been for men's use only, but at this time, it could be enjoyed by women as well.

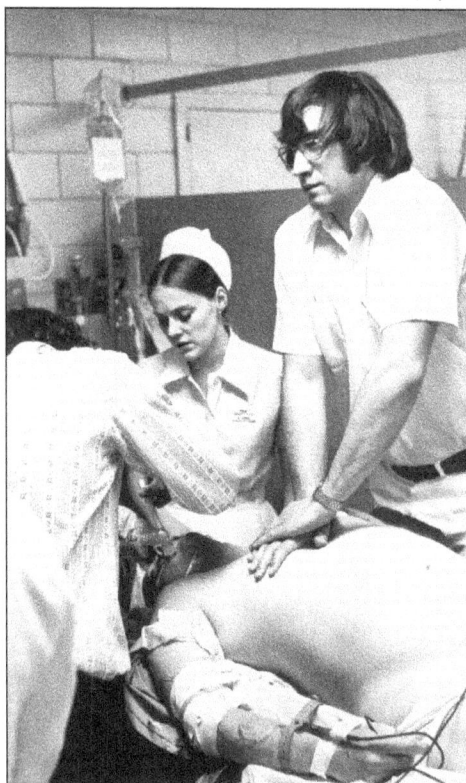

THE EMERGENCY ROOM. In 1982, AMCH was designated as New York's first regional trauma center by the Regional Emergency Medical Organization (REMO) to serve six surrounding counties. In the emergency room, students learned the importance of speed, wise decision making, and working as a team. They also gained a greater understanding of the important relationship and interdependence between the hospital and the community's social and welfare agencies.

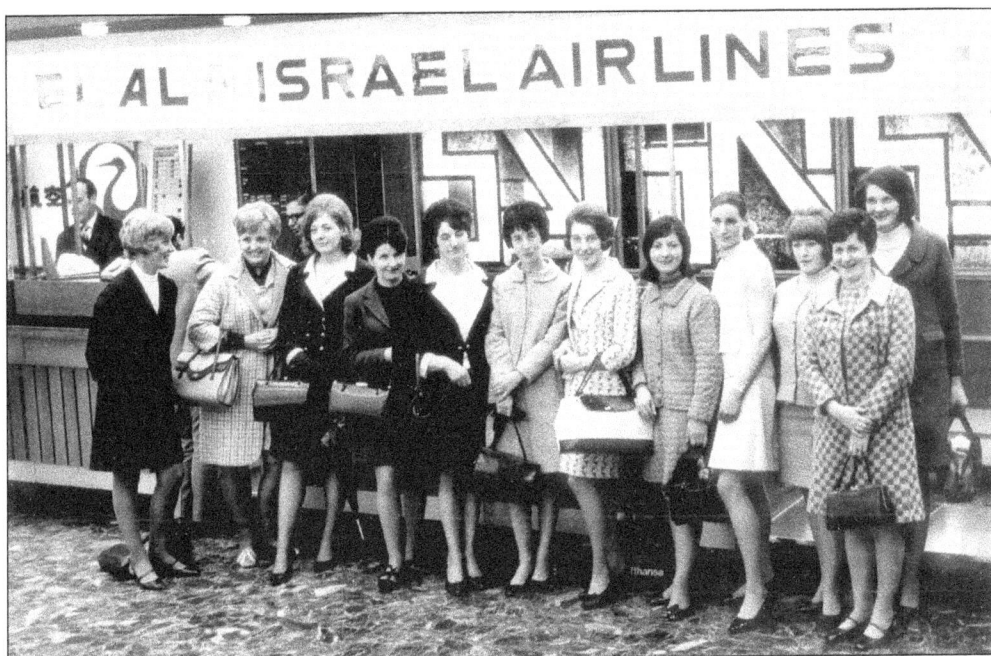

RECRUITING FOREIGN NURSES. In the 1960s, a shortage of nursing staff led to the recruitment of nurses from England, Ghana, Scotland, and other lands. In 1968, this group of nurses awaits departure from Heathrow Airport in England to begin their positions in American hospitals. Seen sixth from the right, Vera Lindsey Frangella, R.N., a nurse midwife, worked in the AMC maternity department until her retirement. (Courtesy Vera Frangella.)

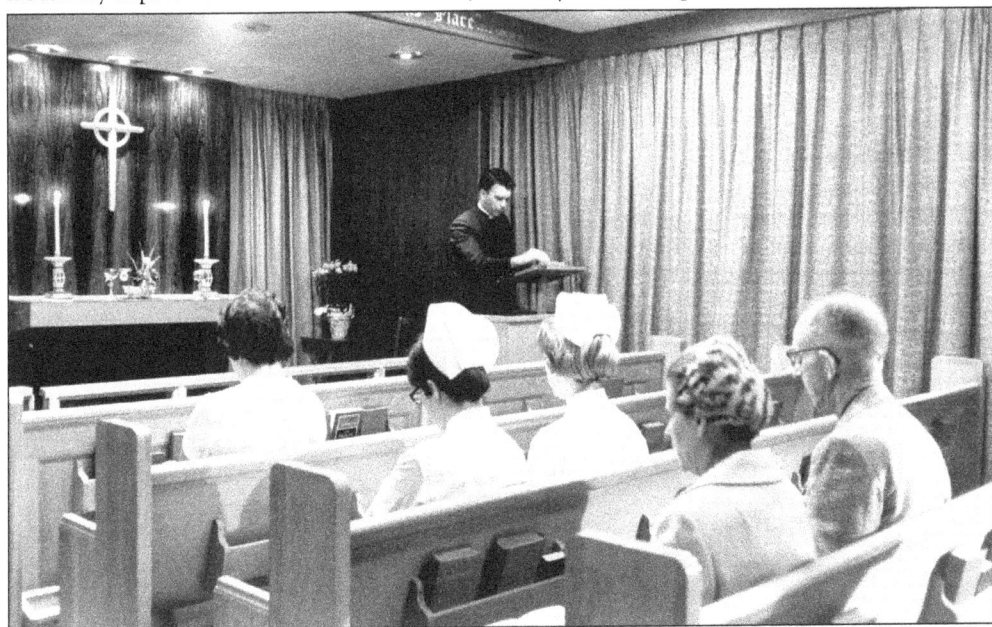

THE KIWANIS MEMORIAL CHAPEL. Located on the second floor of the K Wing, the Kiwanis Memorial Chapel was dedicated in 1954 and was in use until 1991. The new Marcelle Chapel, located on D2 and dedicated in October 1994, was given in memory of Alphonso Marcelle. It is open 24 hours a day for those wishing to pray or meditate.

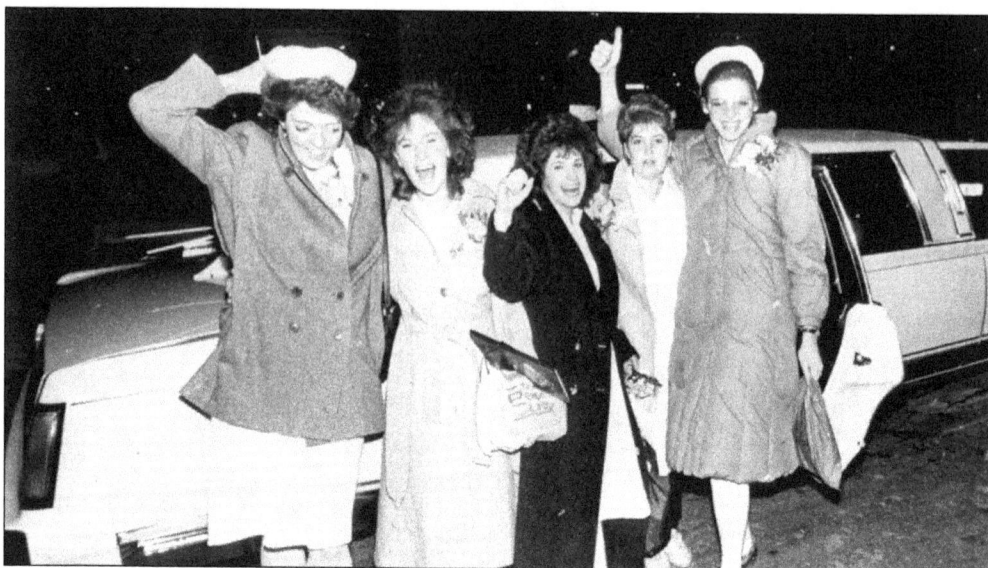

THE WHITE DINNER. Five graduates from the Class of December 1988 celebrate before their limousine ride to the White Dinner. The dinner marked the first time the five wore their white nurses' uniforms. The students are, from left to right, Kim Carney, Jennifer Walsh, Allison Meusberger, Debra Jones, and Audra Bangel.

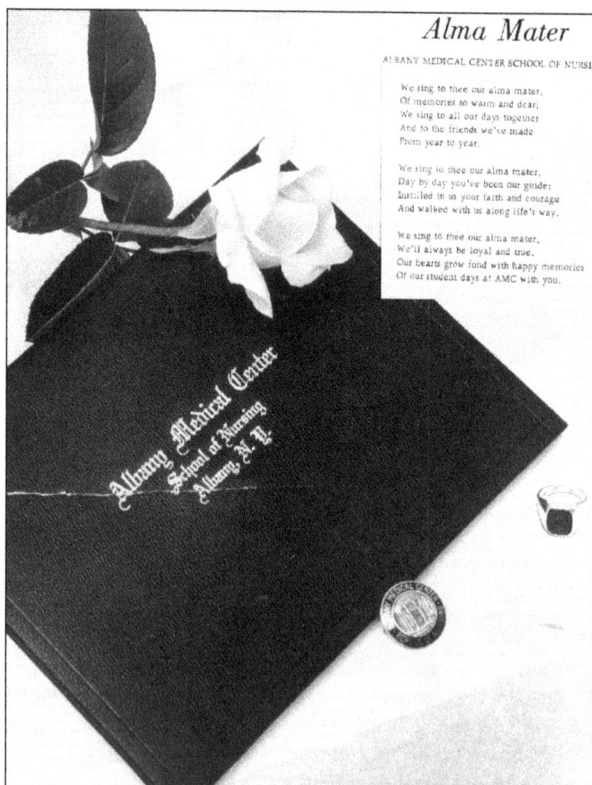

GRADUATION CONFIRMED. The diploma, graduate pin, class ring, rose in open bloom, and alma mater are the symbols of completing the AMCSN program.

MALE NURSES TAKE HONORS. Donald Cameron (left), John Danner (center), and Edward Triebel, Class of Spring 1964, congratulate each other on receiving graduation awards. The Sampson Award for excellence in bedside nursing was given to John Danner and Donald Cameron. The faculty award to a graduating student who has shown the greatest overall personal and professional growth was given to Donald Cameron and John Danner. The alumni award to a graduating student who has excelled in citizenship was given to Edward Triebel.

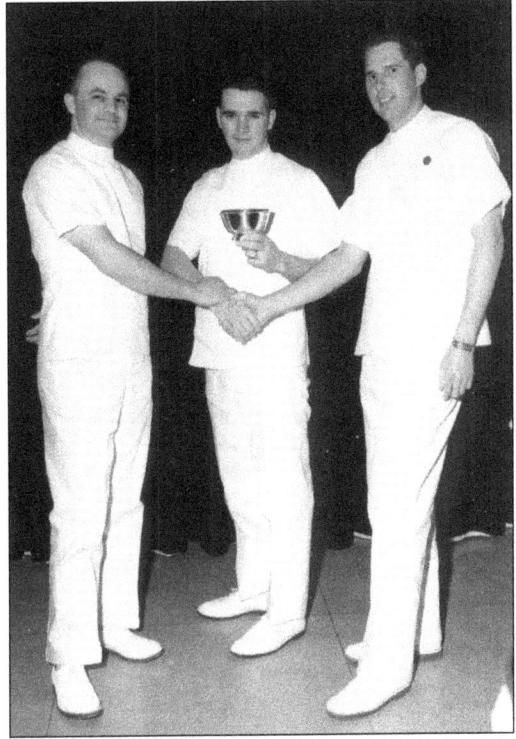

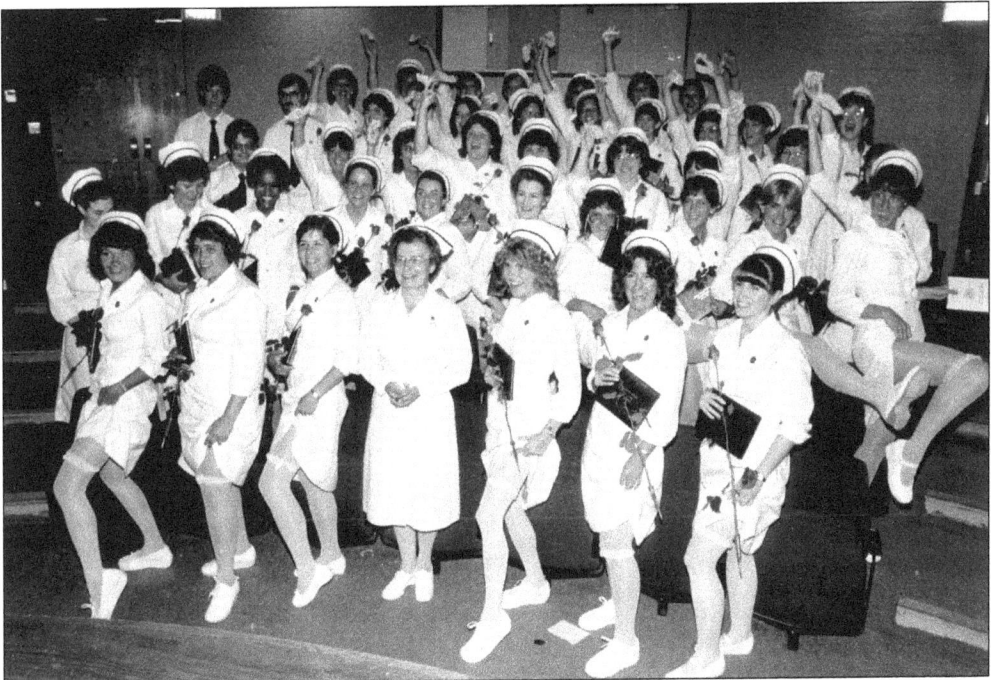

A GRADUATION FLASH, JUNE 1984. Marie Treutler, director of AMCSN from 1972 to 1987, smiles as the graduates, holding their traditional long-stemmed red roses and diplomas, flash white garters in a nontraditional pose.

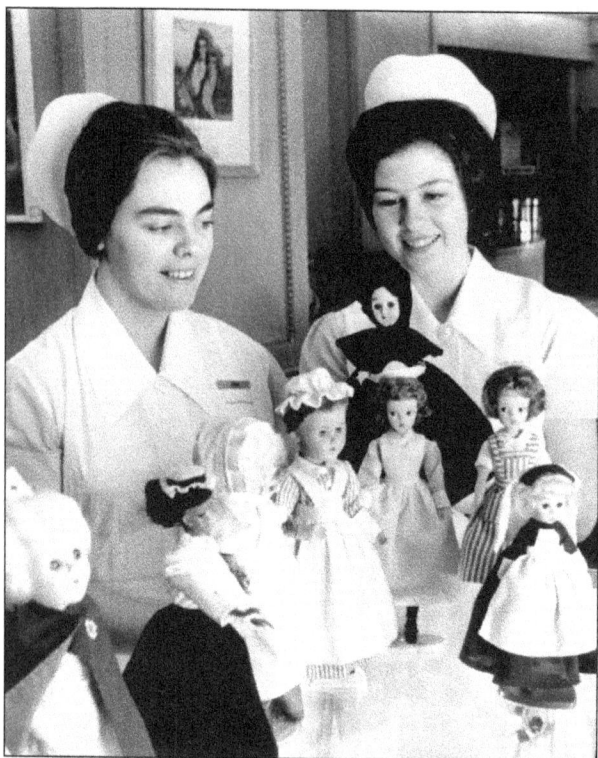

HISTORICAL BEGINNINGS. Elizabeth Boardman Curtin (left) and Lucille Jewett McAllister, Class of Spring 1966, look over an exhibit of dolls depicting nurses throughout history. This project was begun in the history of nursing classes of the early 1960s and has grown to become a popular statement on the wide variety of nursing roles.

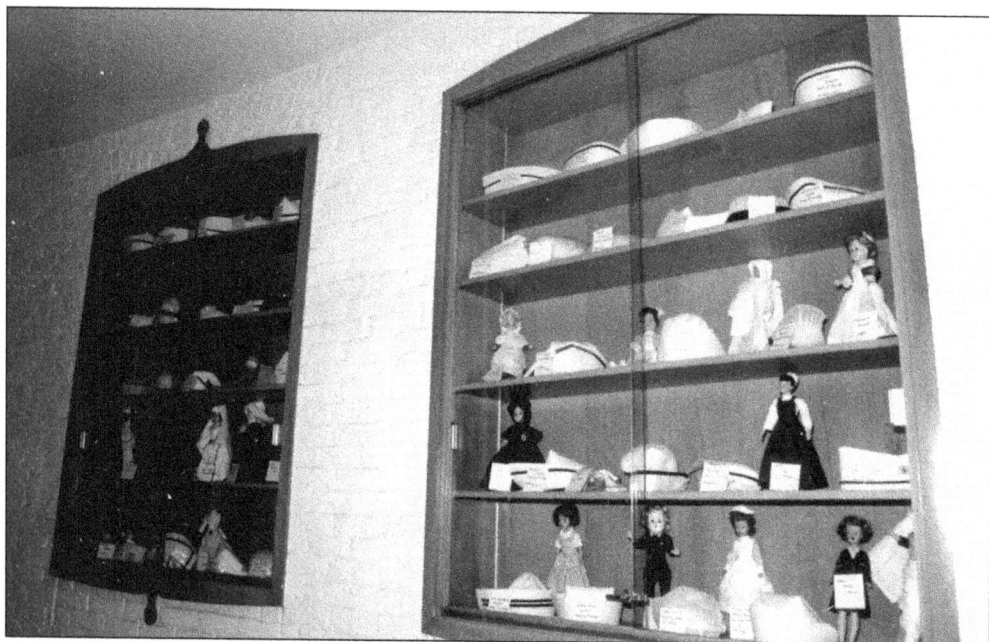

NURSING REMEMBERED. The ramp connecting the third floor of the nurses' residence to the first floor of the hospital became the location for sharing artifacts representing pride in nursing with the public. With the closing of the school, the Alumni Association later moved these items to the Main 4 hallways, now home to many display cases brimming with the schools' memorabilia, as well as graduation and other historical photographs.

Three

INCREASED SPECIALIZATION

IN NURSING PRACTICE

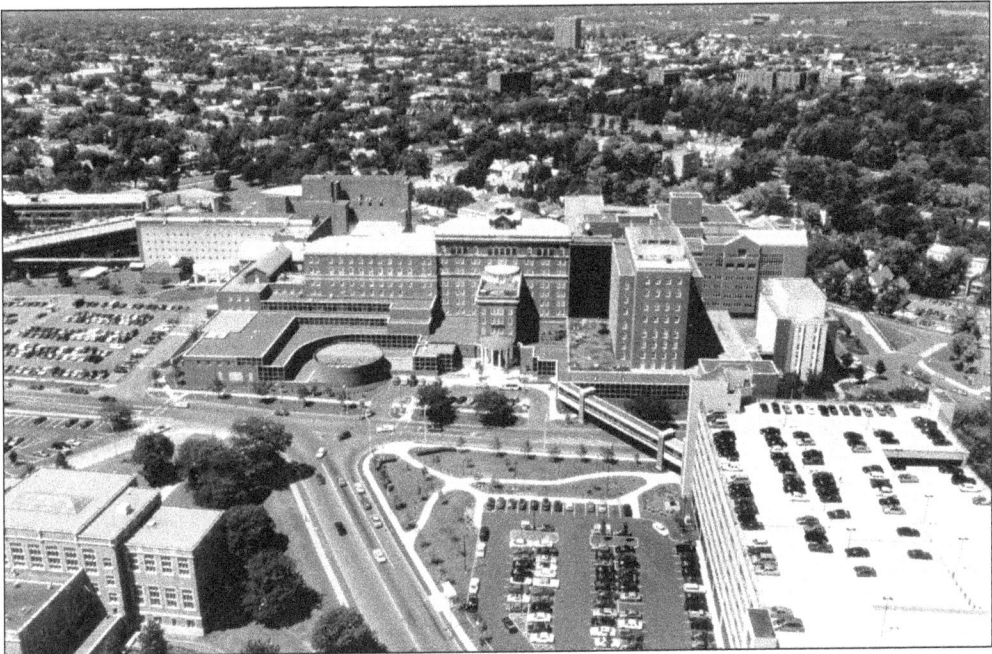

ALBANY MEDICAL CENTER, 2003. Currently, the Albany Medical Center complex includes a new parking garage with an enclosed ramp to the hospital and the David S. Sheridan Magnetic Resonance Imaging Center facing New Scotland Avenue. In 1885, the hospital ministered to a city population of 54,000. Today, Albany Medical Center provides healthcare to over 2.8 million people in 25 counties of northeastern New York and western New England. In celebrating 150 years of service (1849–1999), Albany Medical Center could boast that it was one of America's top 15 major teaching hospitals and top 100 hospitals overall. It is a regional leader in trauma, neurological, perinatal, AIDS, cardiac, cancer, and pediatric care and home to the region's only kidney, pancreas, and bone marrow transplant programs.

Nursing at Albany Medical Center has been a magnificent epic of service and professional development. From the founding days to current practice, nurses have evolved into well-educated and highly trained patient advocates. As staff at an academic health sciences center, nurses continue to lead the way in practice, education, and research for nursing in the community.

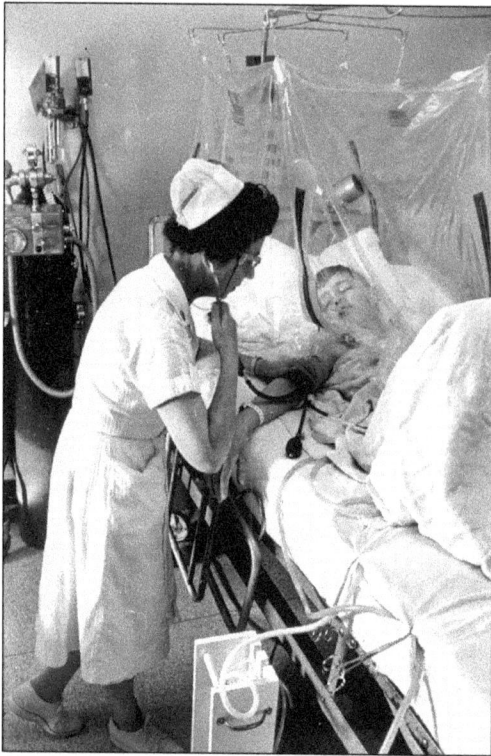

CARDIAC CARE. Private duty nurse Mary McCann, R.N., is shown delivering care to a child in a room designated for pediatric cardiac care. The center's first open-heart surgery on a child in New York State was performed here in 1957. It was only the second open-heart surgery case performed in the state. Private duty nurses taught by physicians provided care to the sickest hospital patients until intensive care units (ICUs) were opened. The pediatric intensive care unit opened in 1970 and was renovated and expanded in 2001.

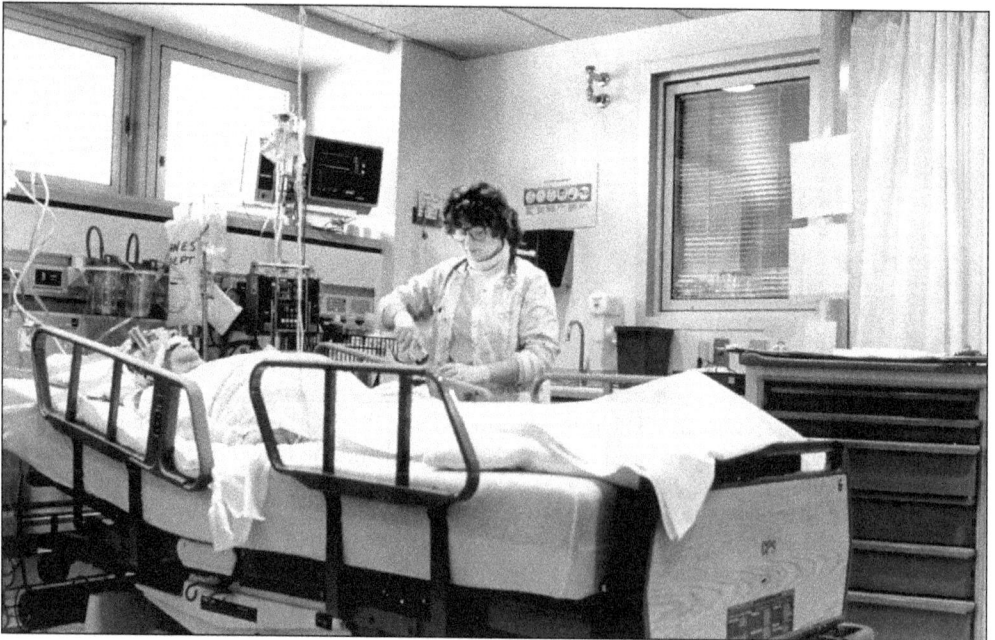

THE CARDIOPULMONARY SURGERY UNIT. The first cardiac care unit opened in 1966, and the nurses' training program for cardiac care began at AMC in 1968 and expanded to include regional nurses in 1970. Robin Belawski, R.N., Class of 1983, cared for one of the first patients in the cardiopulmonary surgery unit that opened in 1991. The first heart transplant was performed at AMC in 2000.

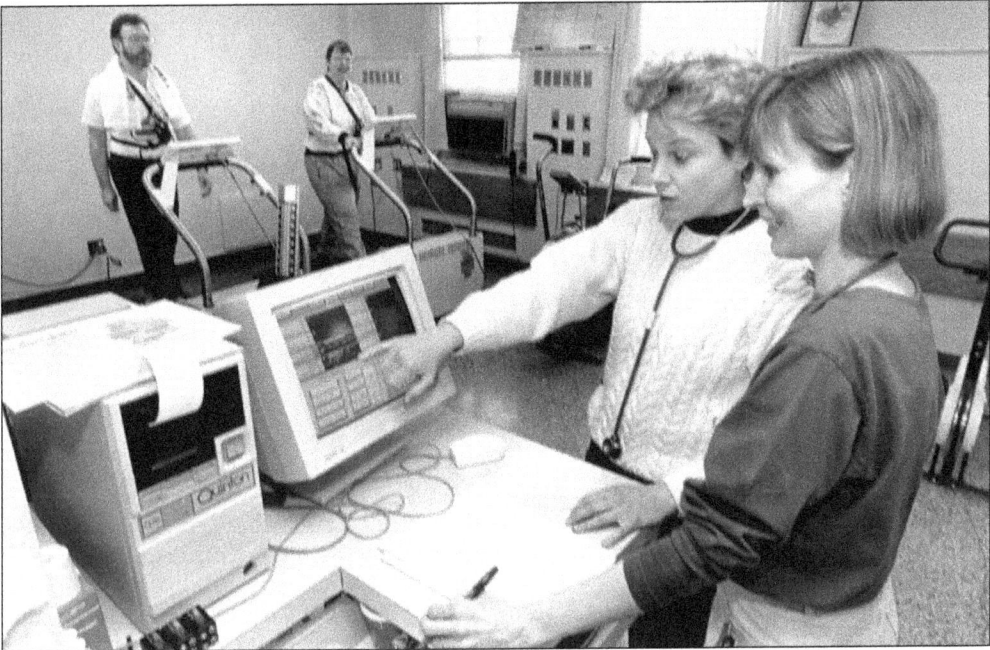

CARDIAC REHABILITATION. Registered nurse Ann Barrett (right) and exercise physiologist Stephanie Spear monitor the progress of patients as they work the treadmills in the cardiac rehabilitation unit. The unit opened on Main 2 in 1991.

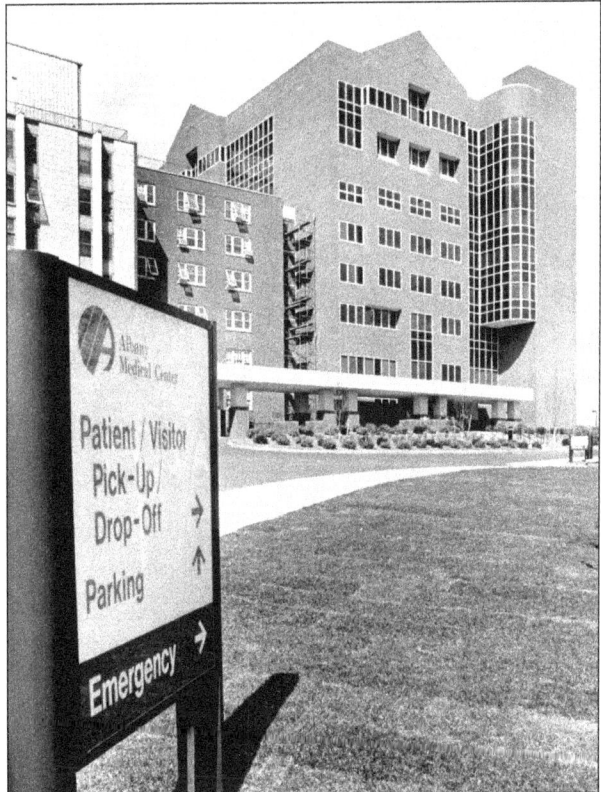

THE PATIENT TOWER OPENS. In 1991, the seven-story patient tower was dedicated. It included a new emergency department, a cardiopulmonary surgery unit, a coronary care unit, surgical and medical intensive care units, a center for cancer and blood disorders, neuroscience and renal transplant units, a birthing center, and a neonatal intensive care unit for the Children's Hospital at Albany Medical Center.

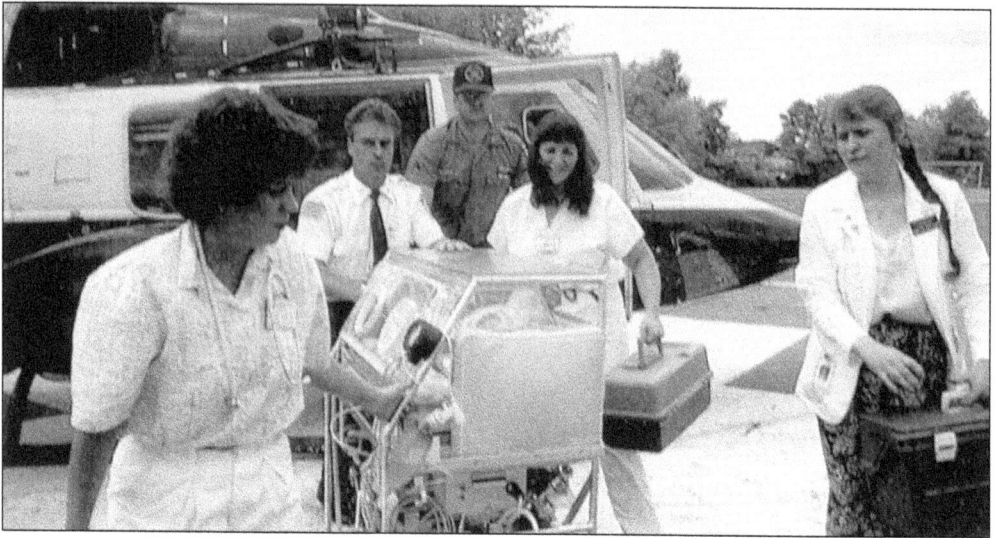

TRANSPORT TEAMS. In 1975, the neonatal transport teams were established to transfer sick newborns from regional hospitals to Albany Medical Center and St. Peter's Hospitals. Throughout the years, medical center staff members have often teamed up with the Air National Guard, New York State Police, and local ambulance squads to provide life-saving air and ground transport for trauma victims or sick newborns.

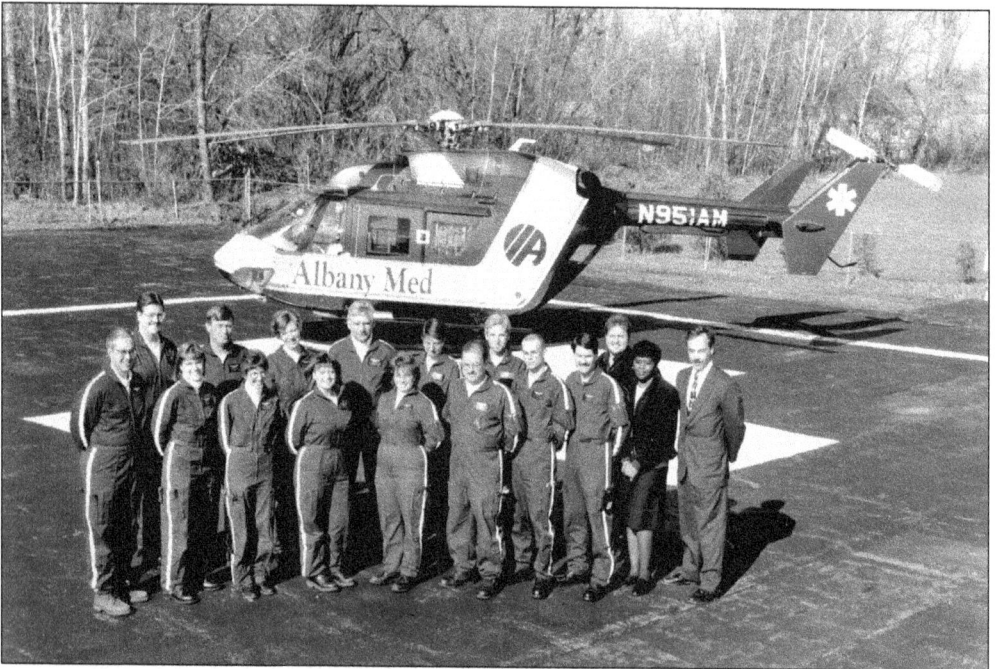

THE MED FLIGHT TEAM, FORMED IN 1966. Members of the Albany Med FLIGHT team are shown in front of a transport helicopter. Albany Medical Center supplies the nurses and paramedics, and Rocky Mountain Holdings LLC supplies the pilots and mechanics. Known as a "flying intensive care unit," the team can be in the air within minutes. An ambulance ride from Newburgh to Albany would take 90 minutes, but by traveling via helicopter the time was cut to 38 minutes.

THE BURN UNIT. The burn unit saved the life of this patient after he suffered burns over 70 percent of his body. Healing occurred with intensive medical and nursing care over a seven-month period. The use of opsonic protein, which theoretically removed abnormal blood platelets, cellular debris, and bacteria, was new at the time and enhanced his recovery. The burn unit was open from 1967 to 1986. Currently, severe burn patients are transported to other burn centers.

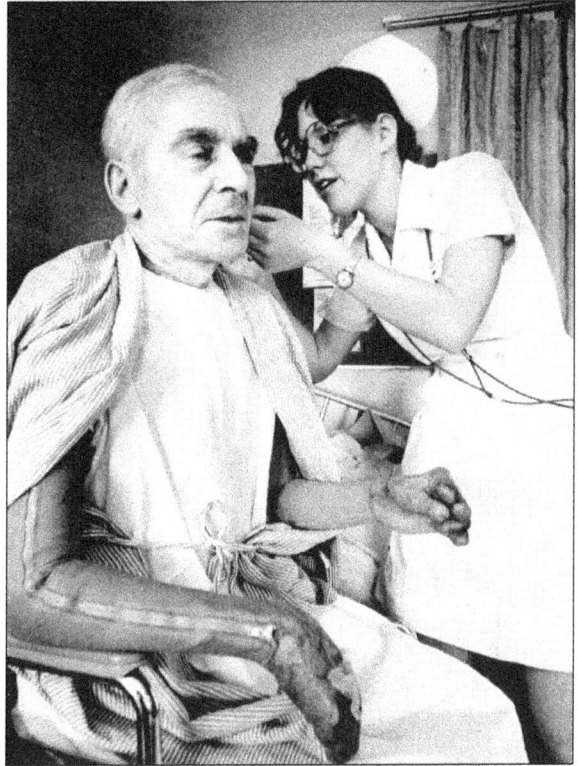

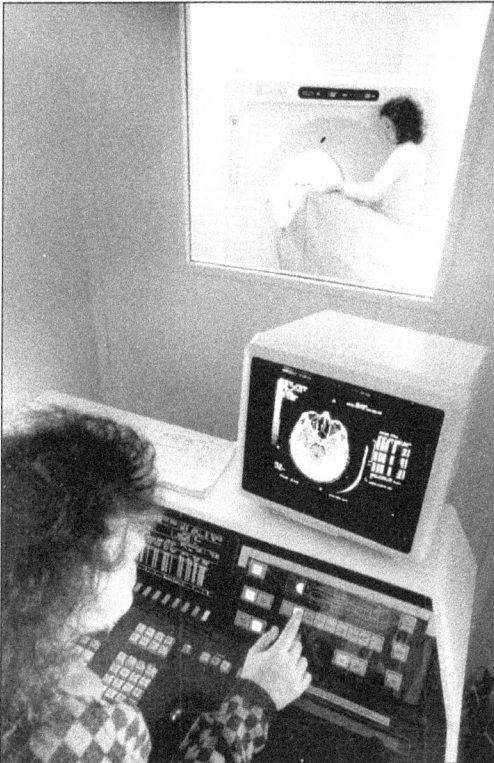

A CAT SCAN FOR THE EMERGENCY ROOM. A decision was made to locate computerized axial tomography, widely known as a CAT scan, in the emergency room. As a result, valuable patient and staff time was saved in determining the extent of injuries to areas of the body, especially to the head, in much greater detail than conventional x-rays could provide.

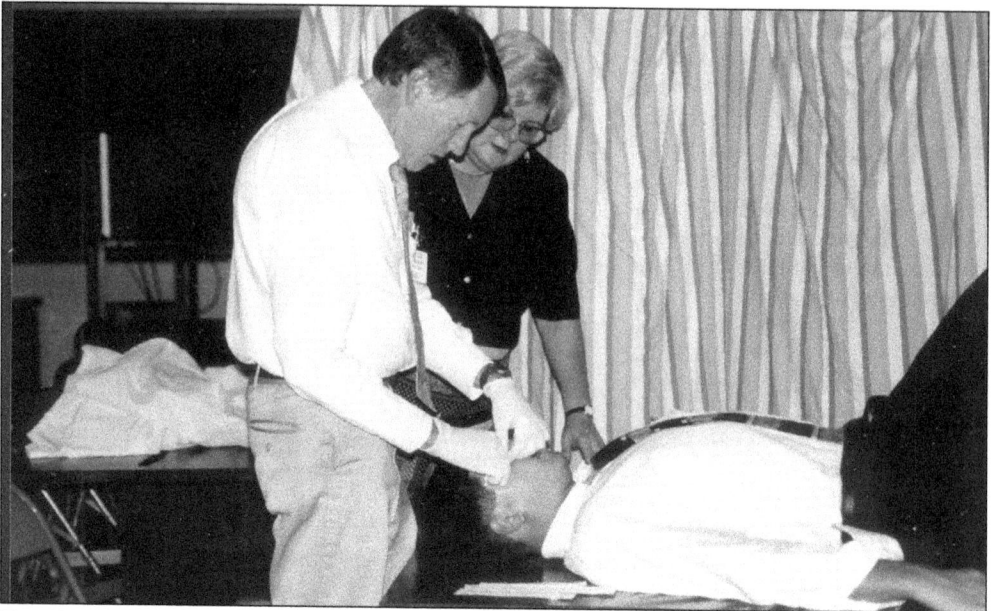

THE PHYSICIAN ASSISTANT PROGRAM. Karen Powles Wolfe, R.N., Class of Fall 1971, the preclinical coordinator for Albany Medical College Center for Physician Assistant Studies, supervises a student during clinical practice. Registered physician assistants-certified are licensed to practice medicine under the supervision of a licensed physician who is not required to be present but must be available by telephone. It is important to know the capabilities of all care team members within Albany Medical Center.

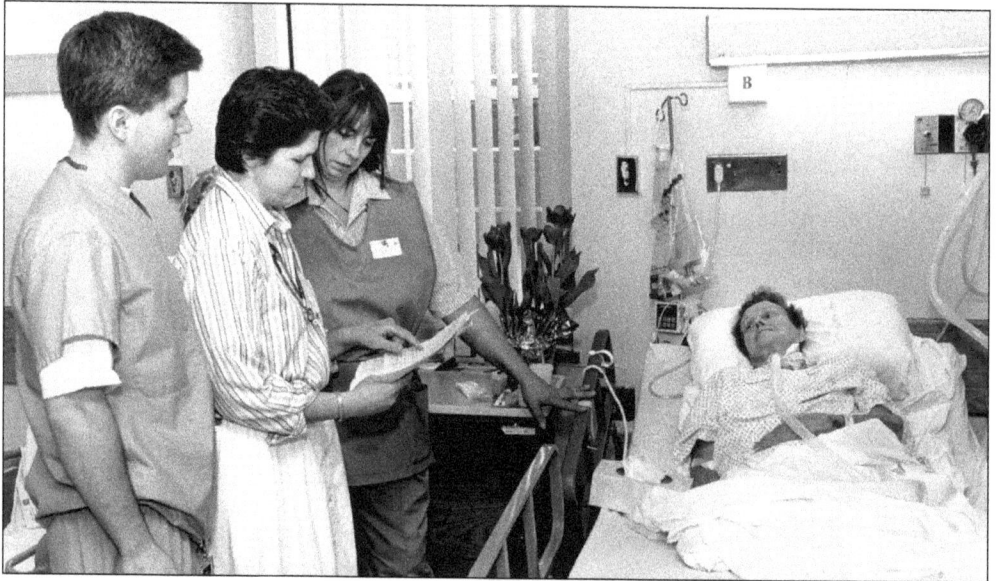

A PATIENT-CENTERED CARE TEAM CONFERENCE. In this patient care model, the registered nurse maintains the role of primary care giver and coordinator of care and is supported by the patient care associate (P.C.A.) with expanded responsibilities beyond that of a nursing assistant. The patient support associate (P.S.A.) attends to the patient's most personal and immediate needs. This team approach gives the registered nurse time for the nursing tasks of care planning, patient education, and discharge preparations.

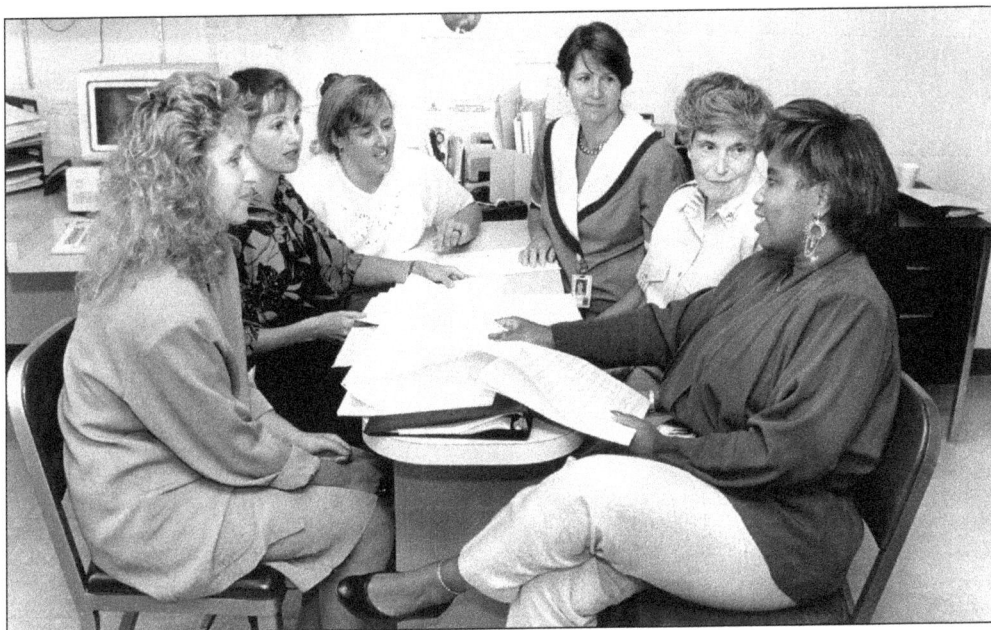

THE ALTERNATE LEVEL OF CARE TEAM. The team works quickly and efficiently to place patients who no longer need acute care into alternate care settings based on health, financial status, special needs, family support, and location. Team members shown here are, from left to right, Pam Werner, B.S.W., a social worker; Kathy Taylor, a referral coordinator; Joyce Ross, R.N., a discharge planner; Jane Metzger, who works in utilization management; Sr. Lucille Theroux, C.S.J., who works in pastoral care; and Sharon Jones, B.S.W., a social worker.

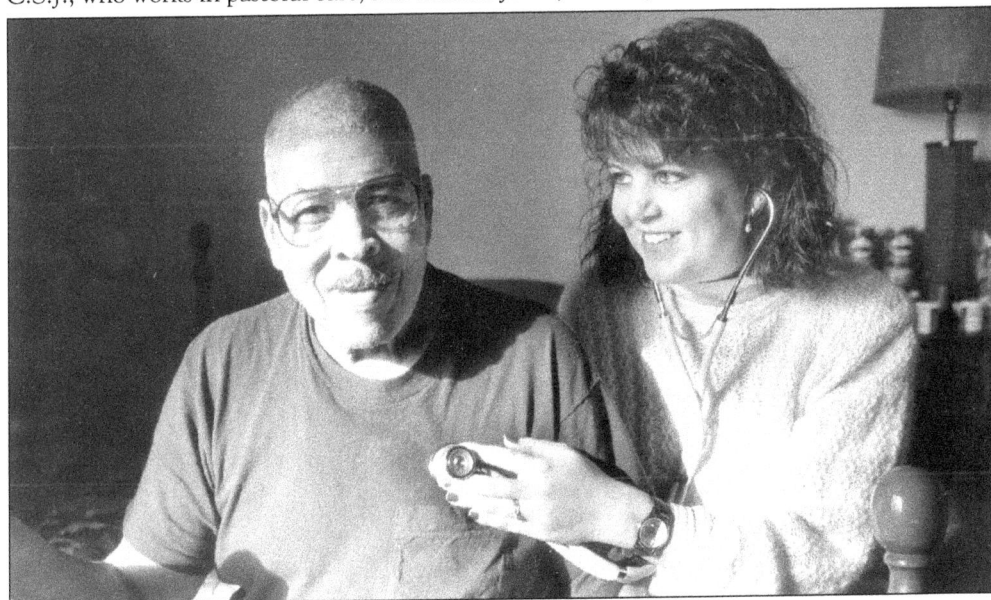

A VISITING NURSE, C. 1997. Visiting nurse Sue Farrell, R.N., helps a diabetic patient manage his illness at his apartment. In 1996, as care moved from hospital to home, Albany Medical Center formed an alliance with the Visiting Nurse Association of Albany in developing home-care programs that provide less duplication and more formal lines of communication for accessing services.

109

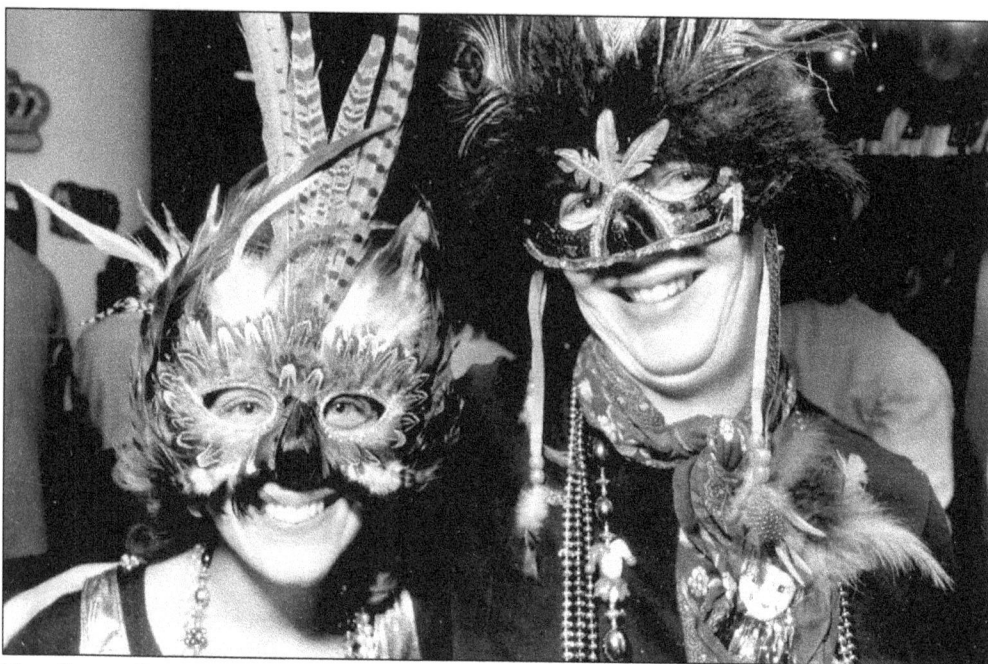

THE JOINT COMMISSION ON ACCREDITATION OF HEALTH CARE ORGANIZATIONS (JCAHO) MARDI GRAS. Jackie Pappalardi, R.N. (left), of environmental health and safety, and Karen Houston, R.N. (right), of quality management, used humor and fun during a Mardi Gras celebration to educate staff about JCAHO standards. During that 1997 JCAHO visit, Albany Medical Center received a rating of 98 points out of a possible 100, the highest rating JCAHO had ever awarded.

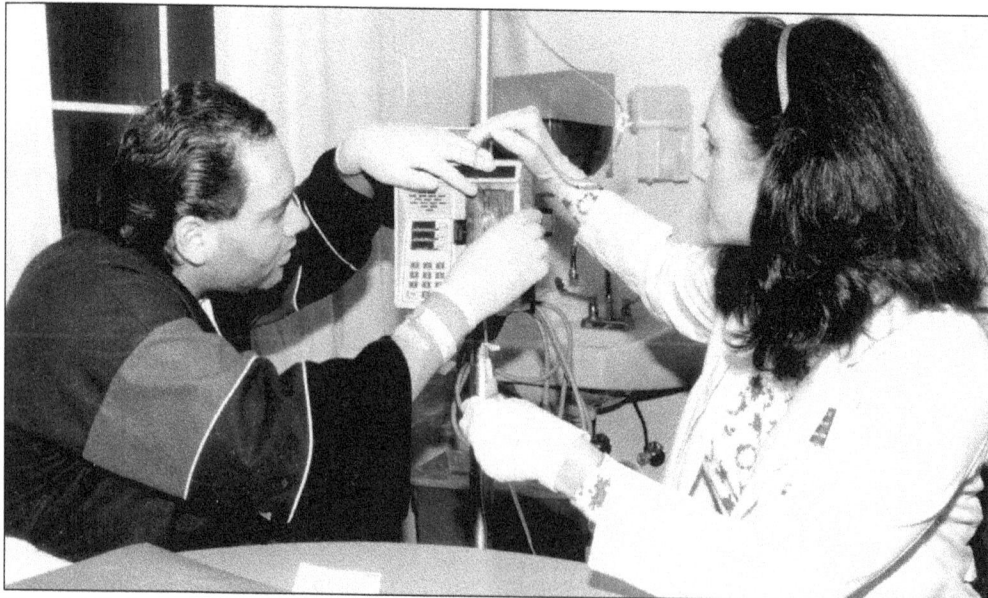

THE 1992 LEARNING CENTER. Nurse educator Kathy Allen, R.N., teaches a patient with a kidney transplant how to operate the intravenous pump he will need to use at home following his hospital stay. Family members and home-care support agencies that provide medications and equipment may also be involved in the individualized teaching plan.

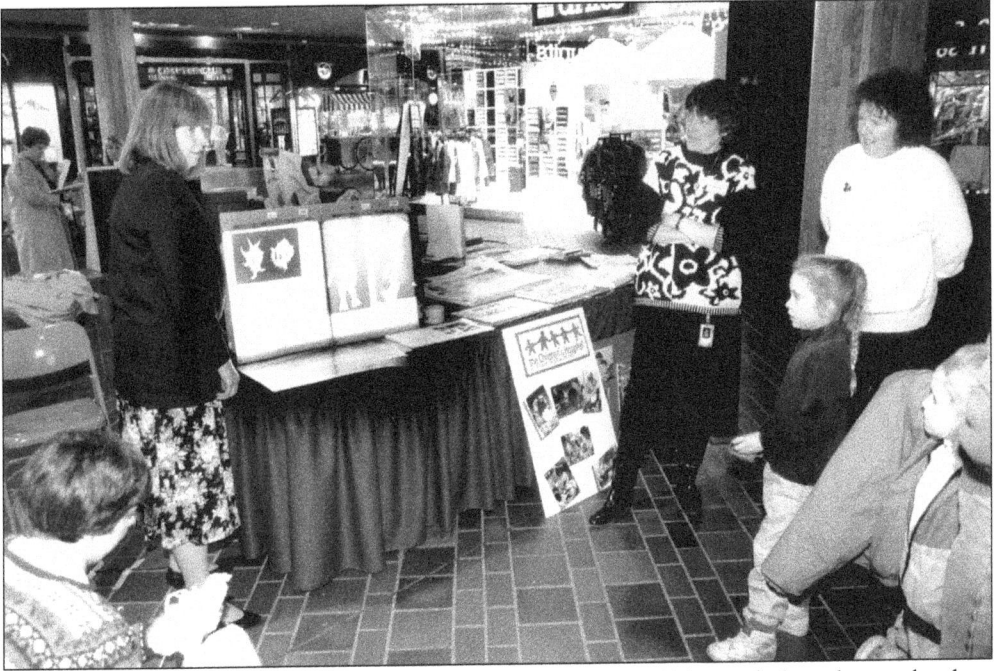

COMMUNITY EDUCATION. Shoppers at Albany's Crossgates Mall learned about hospitals when representatives of the Children's Hospital at Albany Medical Center presented a health fair in conjunction with National Children and Hospital Week. Hospital staff members and young shoppers listen and watch as Elaine Larson DiSieno, R.N., Class of Fall 1974, explains how x-ray films are read.

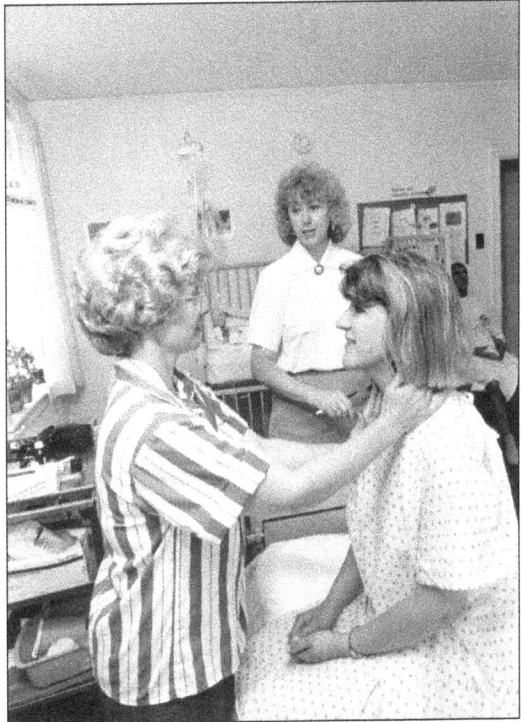

PROJECT LEARN. Project LEARN (Learning, Experience, Assessment, Resources, and Networking) has been a collaborative initiative between Albany Medical Center and the nursing program at Excelsior (Regents) College since 1987. The mission is to provide a unique and alternative path to college education for employees interested in pursuing degrees in nursing. Excelsior College provides an alternative to traditional campus-based programs. Degree programs were later expanded to include business, liberal arts, and technical training.

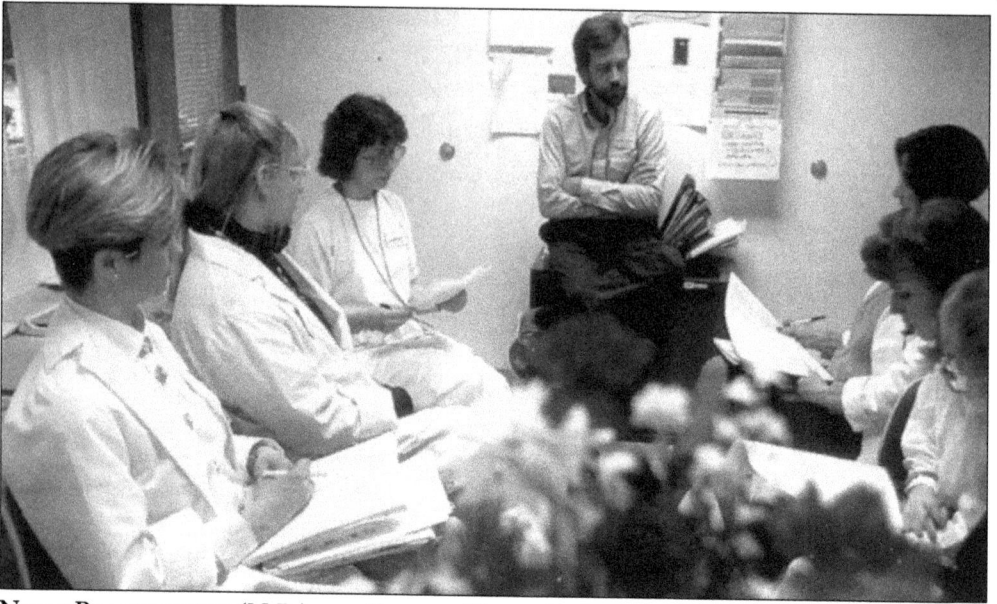

Nurse Practitioners (N.P.) and Clinical Nurse Specialists (C.N.S.). A nurse practitioner program was established at Albany Medical College in 1971. The role of advance practice nurses has expanded and evolved with the hiring of the first clinical nurse specialists in 1979. Within the hospital setting, clinical nurse specialists and nurse practitioners have contributed significantly to quality patient care. Pictured here, Stephen Jones, M.S., R.N. Certified, C.N.S/N.P., is leading multidisciplinary patient care rounds.

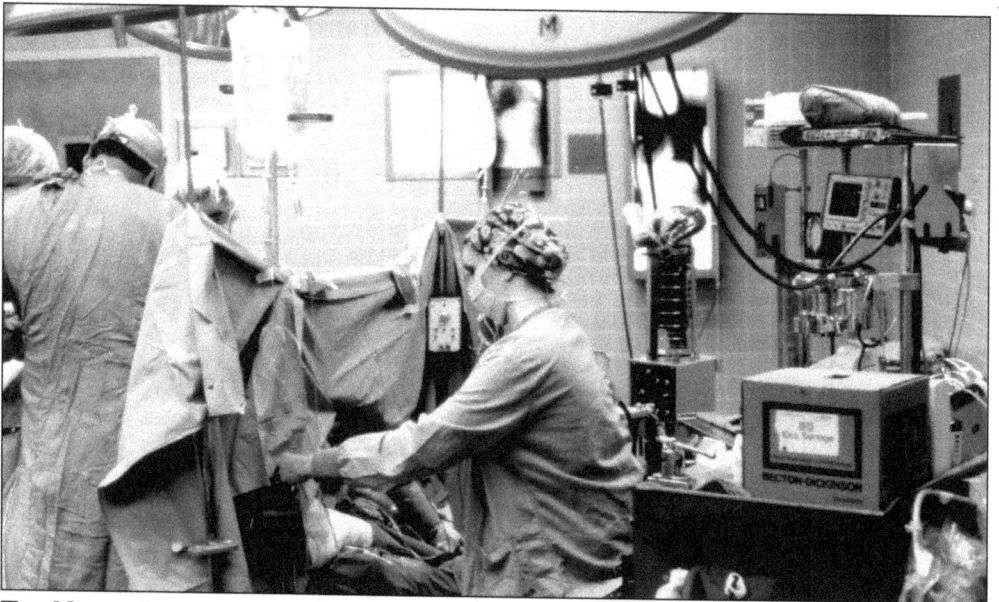

The Nurse Anesthesiology Program. The nurse anesthesiology program was established at Albany Medical Center (AMC) in July 1951. A master's degree program was implemented in 1986. After certification, nurse anesthetists at AMC become members of the anesthesia care team, which is coordinated by an attending anesthesiologist. These professionals provide anesthesia to patients who undergo surgical, diagnostic radiology, or psychiatric procedures.

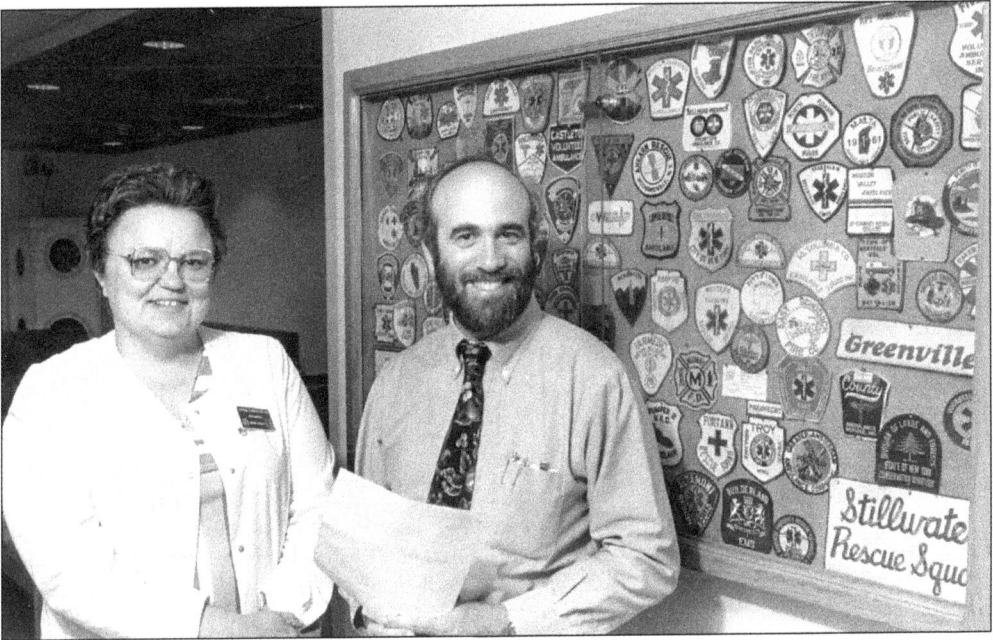

EMERGENCY EXCELLENCE. In 1992, Johanna Franz Flanigan, R.N., Class of Fall 1969, the nurse manager of the emergency department, and Dr. Dan Mayer, an emergency department physician, were recognized by the Regional Emergency Medical Organization (REMO). Flanigan was presented with the REMO Emergency Medical Services Leadership Award, and Mayer was named emergency physician of the year. As emergency medicine outreach coordinator from 1994 to 2003, Flanigan served as liaison between local emergency medical services and the hospital and also coordinated educational activities for them.

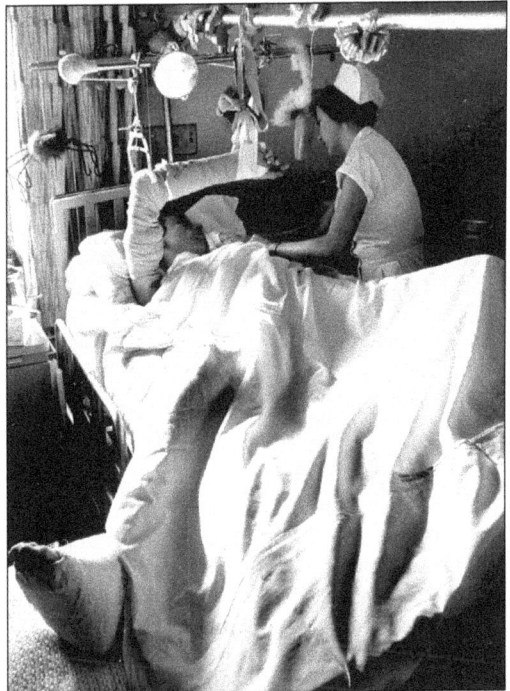

ORTHOPEDIC NURSING. Equipment used in orthopedic nursing can be intimidating to patients and families. The outcome of procedures can determine future mobility and functions that can affect the rest of their lives. As well as understanding the physics of the orthopedic equipment, nurses must be aware of the interaction of physical needs and emotional responses and the potential financial impact in the rehabilitation process.

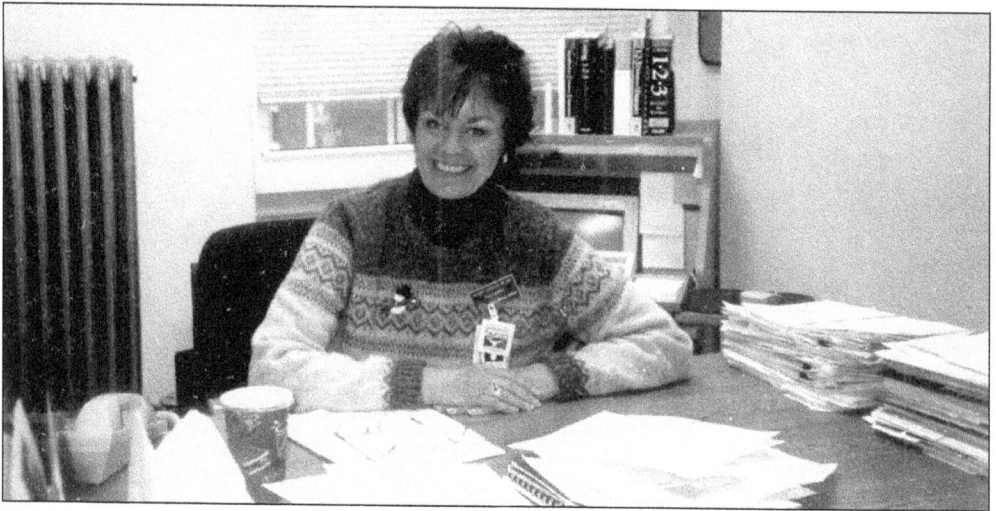

FISCAL ADMINISTRATION. In the data management and informatics world, nurses work in many areas, including information and quality management and health information services. Shown here is Barbara Simpson Leafer, R.N., Class of Spring 1964, an expert in software and spreadsheet design who develops, monitors, and evaluates productivity, budget plans, and data within patient care services for the inpatient units.

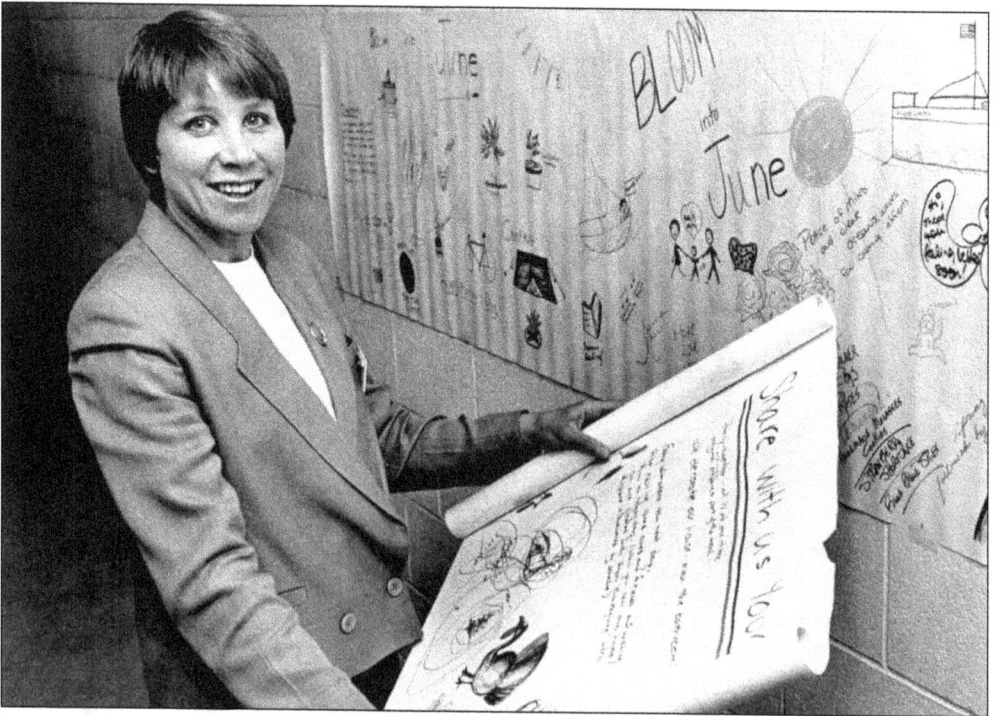

LAUGHTER IS THE BEST MEDICINE. When people laugh together, they work together better and handle stress more easily. Lisa Faist-Stanton, M.S., R.N., a clinical nurse specialist, displays some murals nurses have drawn to break up their routine and release their creativity. She recalls Yellow Day as it was explained to a patient: "Everybody wore yellow to help relieve the day-to-day stress of nurses on the floor. Later with a poker face, that patient presented her nurse with a bedpan full of yellow bananas."

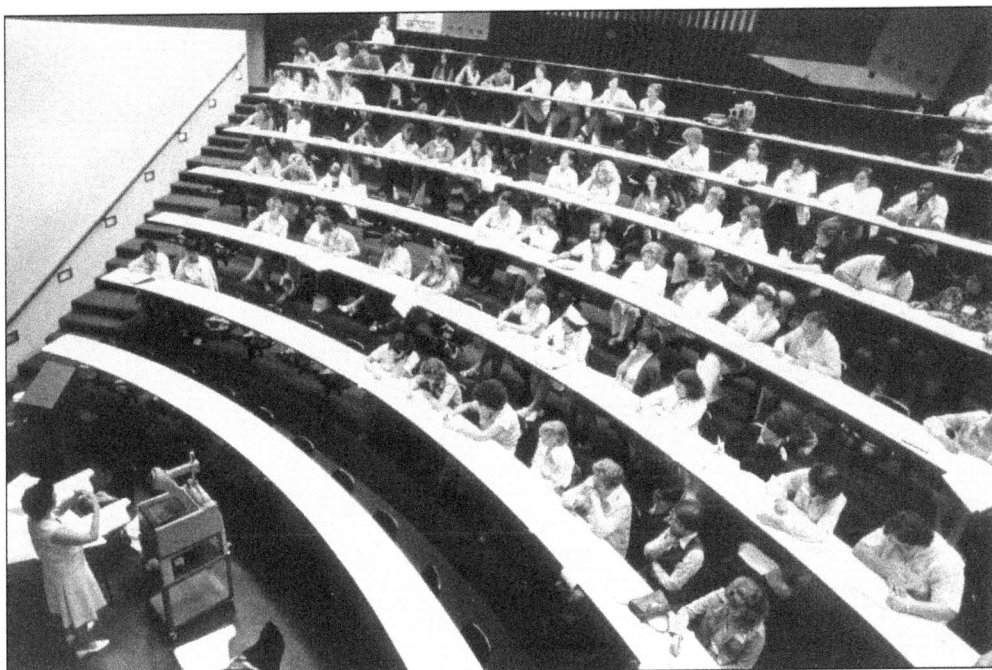

TOGETHER WE LEARN. Multidisciplinary administrative meetings, lectures, and educational programs are frequently held in the ME300 auditorium at Albany Medical College.

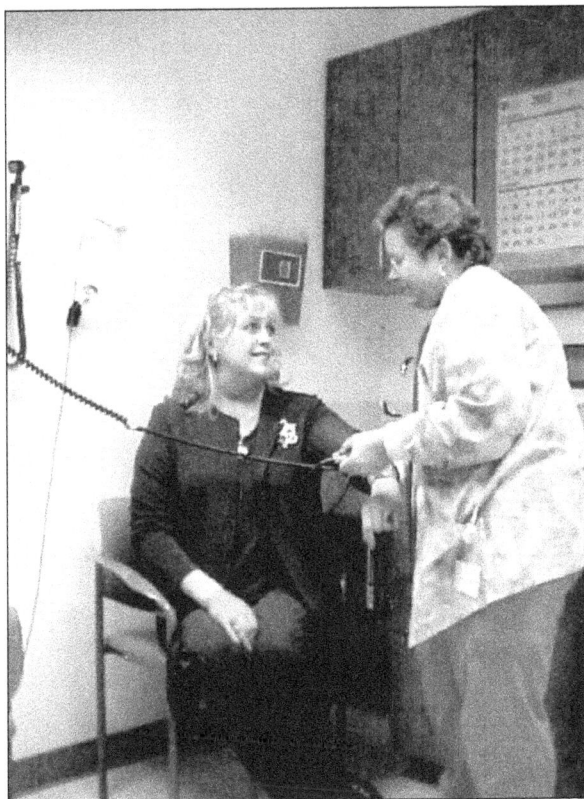

RADIATION ONCOLOGY. Oncology certified nurse Doreen Schrank, B.S., R.N., Class of Fall 1977, begins a nursing assessment for this patient's weekly treatment follow-up visit, which includes checking weight, laboratory values, nutritional status, and side effects from the radiation treatment. Patients are encouraged to maintain as normal a lifestyle as possible. Radiation therapy may be used for the primary modality of cancer treatment, an adjunct therapy, or palliation.

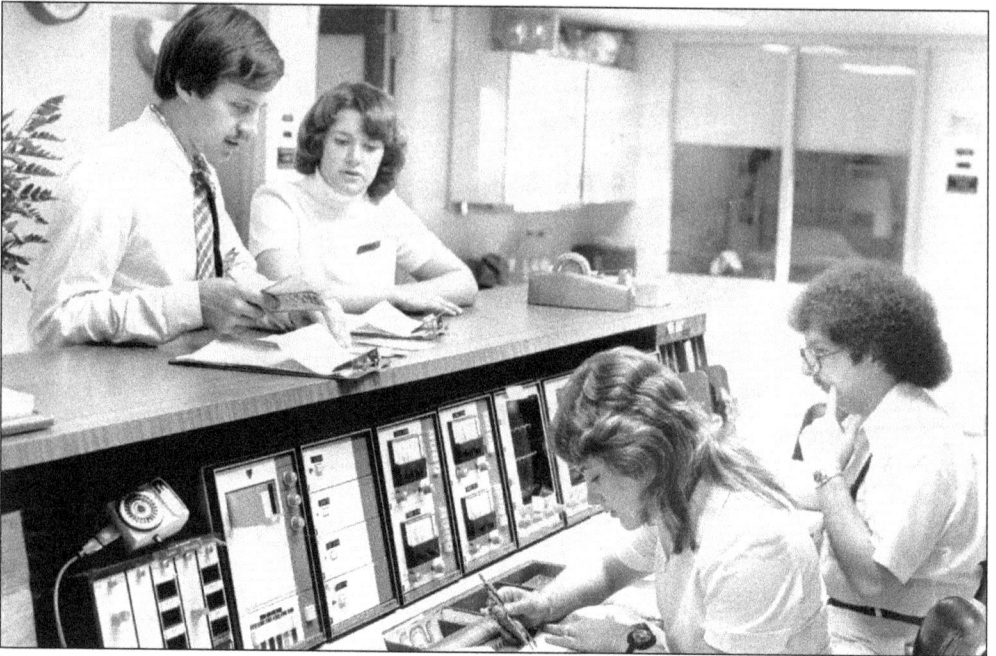

REGISTERED NURSES AND SPECIALIZATION. Nancy Lake-Dahl, R.N., discusses a patient's condition with a physician. Other staff members are shown observing cardiac rhythms at a bank of monitors. Specialization in nursing practice is needed for these positions. Over the years, career ladders have been established to focus on areas of education, management, and clinical practice. Beginning in 1973, ANA certification in one's area of specialty such as pediatrics, obstetrics, administration, and critical care was recognized through national exams.

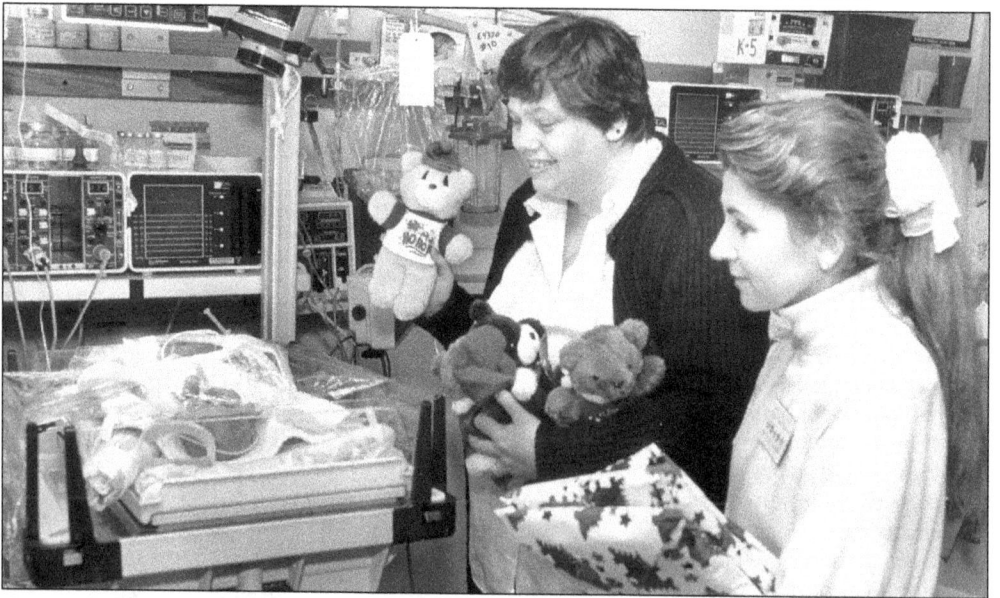

GIFTS TO OUR TINIEST PATIENTS. Pictured here are Sarah Preece of Ballston Spa and Elaine Bobseine Frank, R.N., Class of Spring 1977, a case manager in the neonatal intensive care unit (NICU). Preece donated quilts that she made and bears that she purchased to the babies in the NICU during the holiday season.

THE RONALD MCDONALD HOUSE. The 16-bedroom Ronald McDonald House, at 139 South Lake Avenue, opened in 1982. This was the first upstate home away from home for out-of-town families of hospitalized patients needing nearby lodging and a hot meal at night. Debbie Ross has been the resident house manager since the program began in Albany. Community support and the loose change from the canisters of the 80 regional McDonald's Restaurants assist with the $600,000 annual budget.

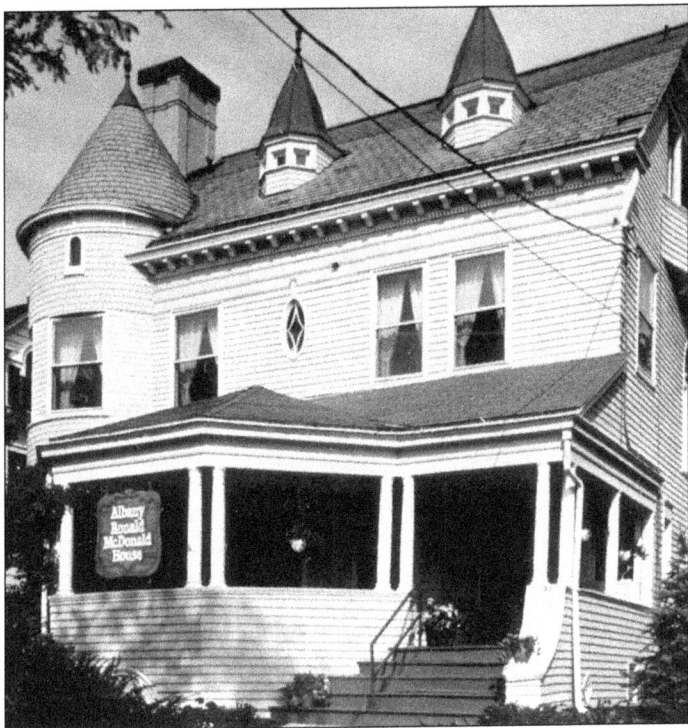

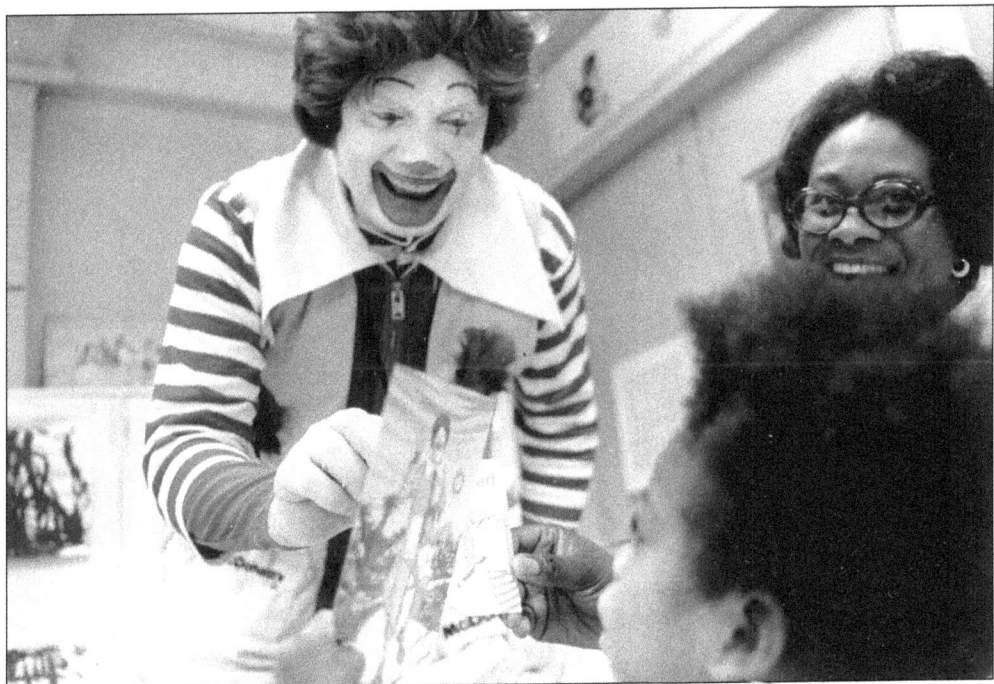

FILLING UP ON LAUGHTER. Ronald McDonald visited patients at Albany Medical Center. Families, staff, and young patients enjoyed the fun.

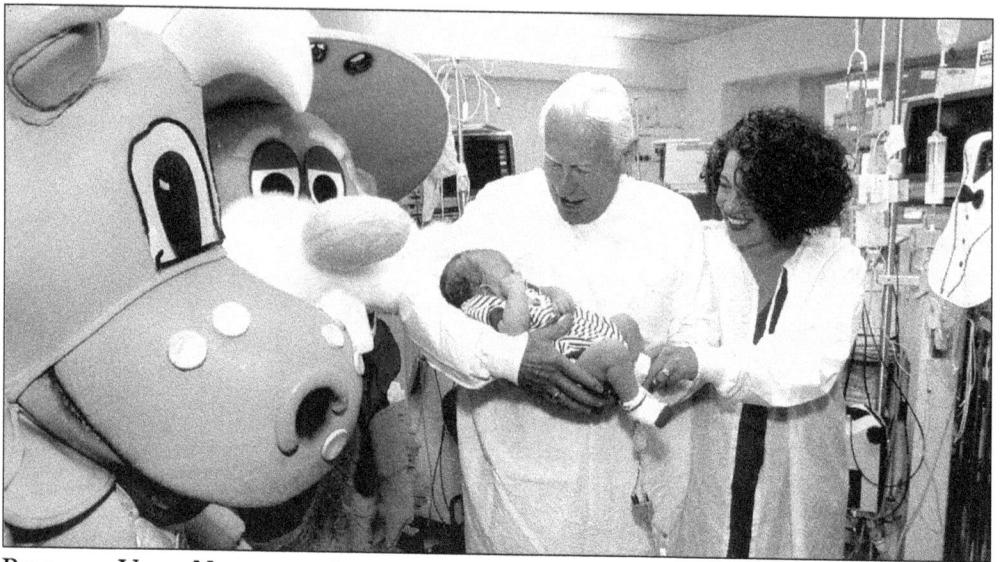

PEDIATRIC UNITS NAMED FOR CHARLES R. WOOD. In 1992, Charles R. Wood, "the Father of the Theme Parks," was honored for his generosity to the Children's Hospital at Albany Medical Center when the inpatient units were officially named the Charles R. Wood Pediatric Inpatient Center. He is also known for his development of an Adirondack summer camp, the Double "H" Hole in the Woods Ranch, where AMCH staff volunteer by providing the children at the camp with medical and nursing care.

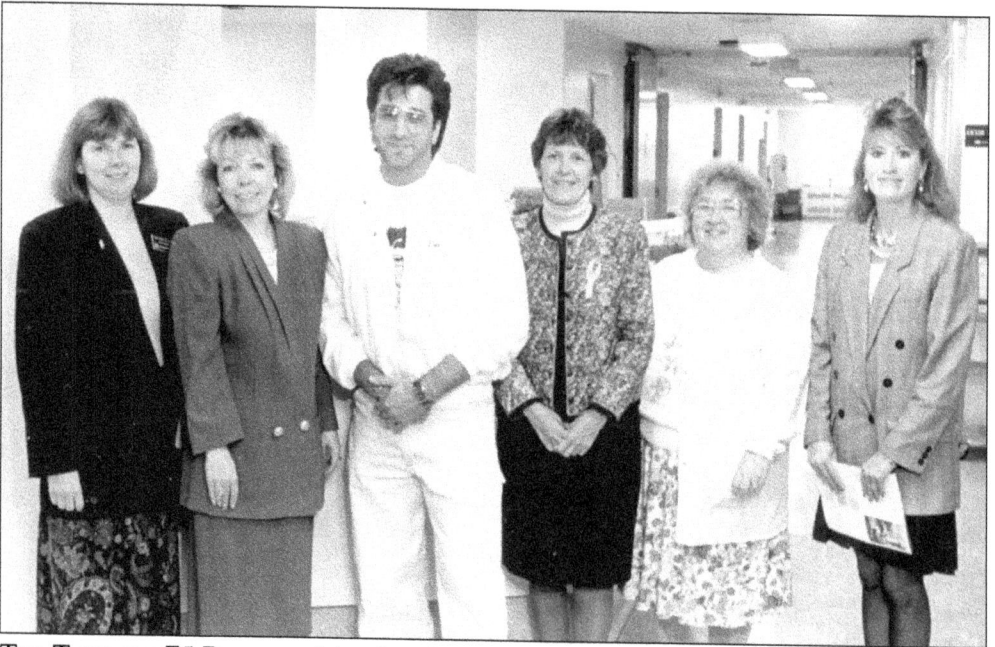

THE TEAM FOR E5 REDESIGN. Mary Lou Brennan, R.N. (not in the photograph), spearheaded the team, shown in a Junior League of Albany project to redesign the women's health unit on E5. Local artists contributed art for the walls. The solarium was provided with home-style furniture, and patient rooms were supplied with floral and designer-print spreads and privacy curtains. They also furnished a staff lounge as well as a meeting room and library for the staff and patients.

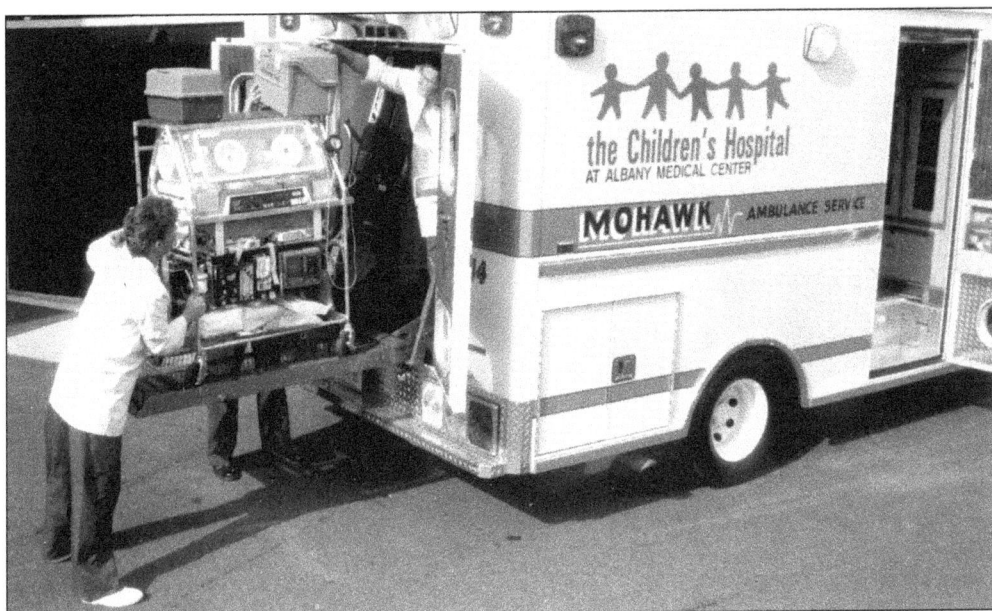

MOHAWK AMBULANCE ADDS THE CHILDREN'S HOSPITAL LOGO. In 1989, Mohawk Ambulance received the exclusive contract for Albany Medical Center's pediatric patients and made the decision to fully equip an ambulance for pediatric or neonatal cases only. The logo of the Children's Hospital at Albany Medical Center on the ambulance makes this identification most clear.

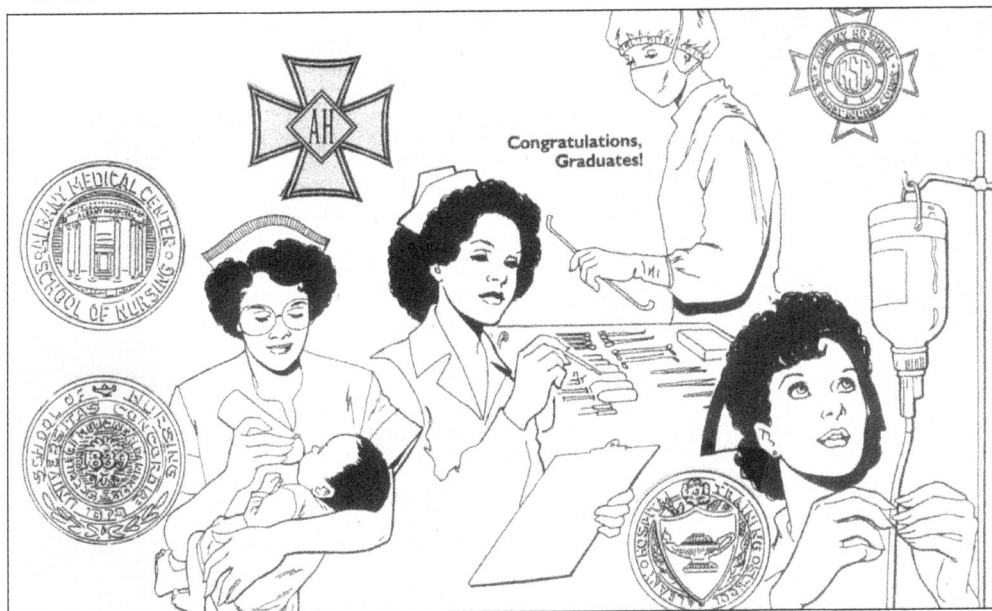

GRADUATION PINS. Graduation pins of the Albany Medical Center Schools of Nursing Alumni Association are, appearing clockwise, the Albany Medical Center School of Nursing (1955–1989); the Albany Hospital Training School for Nurses (1897–1924); the U.S. Cadet Nurse Corps affiliated with Russell Sage College and Albany Hospital (1942–1947); the Albany Hospital Training School for Nurses (1925–1937); and the Union University School of Nursing (1945–1957).

119

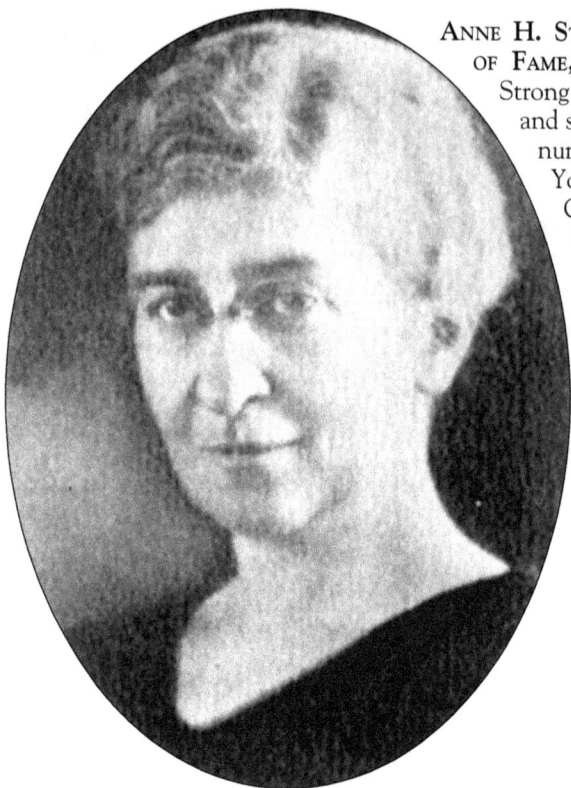

ANNE H. STRONG INDUCTED INTO NURSING HALL OF FAME, 1984. As a graduate, Anne Hervey Strong, R.N., Class of 1906, was an instructor and supervisor at Albany Hospital and a staff nurse at the Henry Street Settlement in New York City. She attended Teachers College, Columbia University, and subsequently became an instructor in public health there. She became the first director of Simmons College School of Public Health Nursing, a post she held until her death in 1925.

JANN DOWNING LUNIEWSKI, M.S., R.N., CLASS OF SPRING 1966. James J. Barba, president, chief executive officer, and chairman of the board of directors, presents Jann Luniewski with the Pillars Award. The center's highest honor pays tribute to individuals who embody the principles of excellence, longtime service, and dedication to the center. Luniewski was also named employee of the year in 1992.

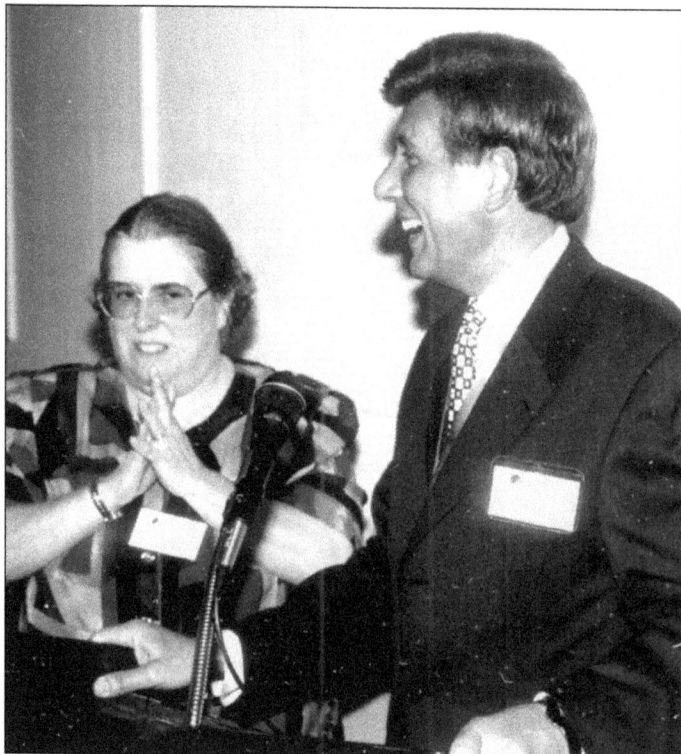

120

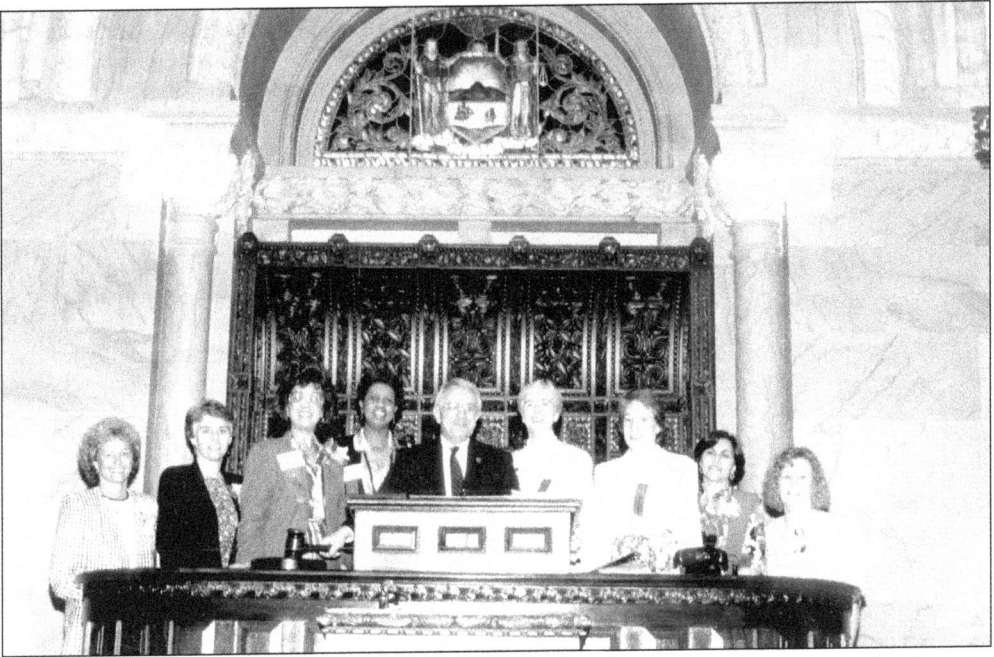

PATRICIA COFFEY, M.S., R.N., C.N.S, FETED. In 1992, clinical nurse specialist Patricia Coffey, second from the left, and seven other nominees are shown at the state capitol with Sen. Tarky Lombardi. They earned the honor of being named regional finalists in the state legislature's Nurse of Distinction Award. Clinical nurse specialist Coffey was selected by the medical center for her work in expanding patient education in obstetrics, gynecology, family planning, and pediatrics.

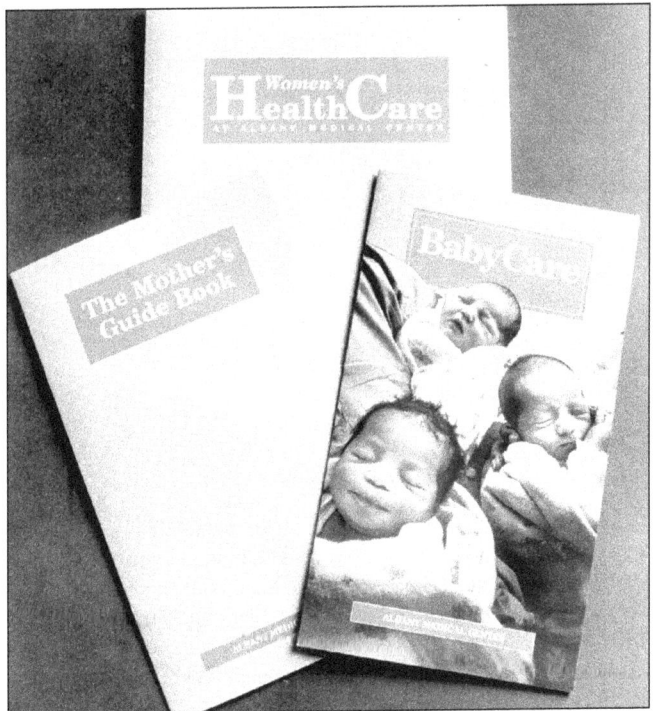

THREE BOOKLETS AWARDED TOP HONOR. Three booklets published by the Albany Medical Center Department of Women and Children won a top 10 award in 1991 from the Food and Drug Administration and the National Coalition for Consumer Education. Authors of the booklets were Lauren Albright, M.S., R.N., N.P.; Patricia Coffey; Jeanne Elisha, M.S., R.N., C.N.S; and Maureen Kimball, B.S.N., R.N.

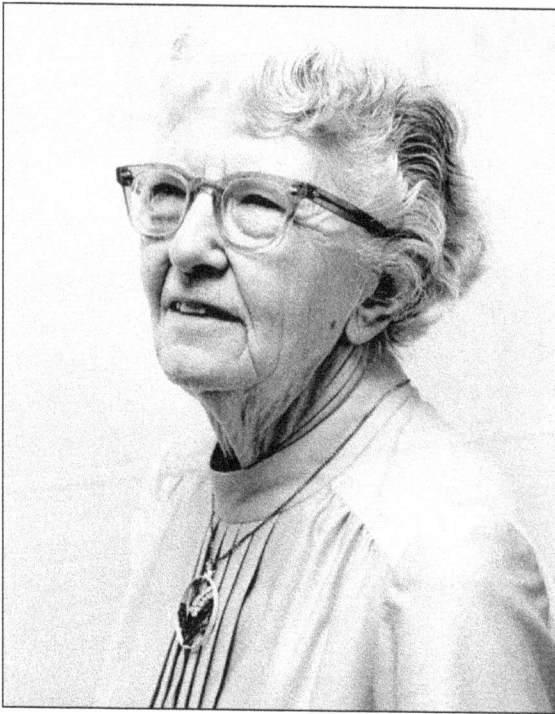

LOUISE DENISON, R.N., CLASS OF 1928. The amount of research Louise Denison did on the history of the nursing schools at Albany Medical Center was monumental. In a tribute of her work, her notes were typed for inclusion in the Alumni Association's archival material and used in this history. Alumni reunions, first instituted by Denison in 1963, have been a highlight each year, especially for the honored five-year anniversary classes.

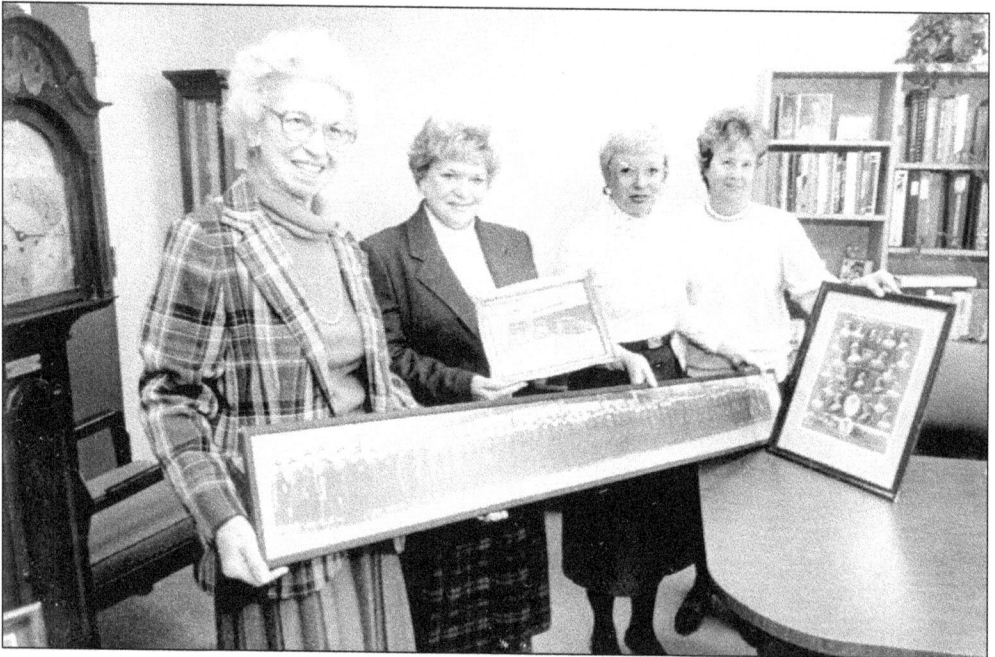

THE ALUMNI ASSOCIATION FINDS PICTURES. From left to right, registered nurses Verna Rolf, Janet Gardner, Sandra Scudder, and Audrey Finlayson Woolsey, Class of 1949, hold photographs discovered while researching material for the Alumni Association's video *Alumni Remembrances 1897–1989.* In 1988, a New York State resolution was received by alumni president Janet Gardner commemorating the closing of AMCSN and preserving the history of the nursing schools through a video.

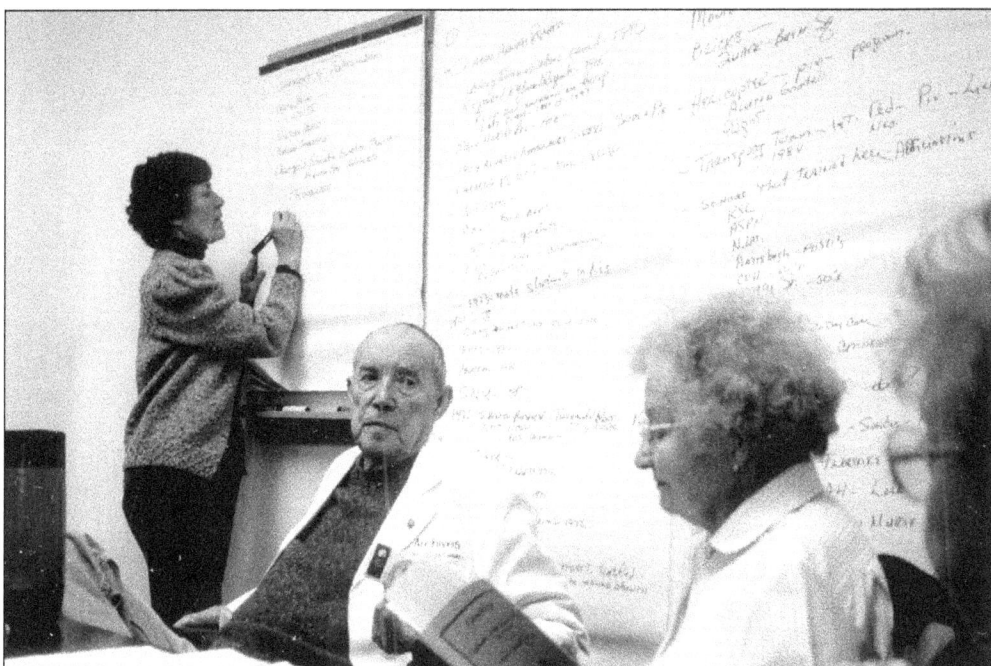

A History of Nursing Exhibit Work Session. From left to right are Elsie Lingelbach Whiting, R.N., Class of 1955, the Alumni Association president; Rue Moore, the medical center archivist; Marie Treutler, the third director of AMCSN; and Audrey Woolsey in a work session for the permanent nursing history exhibit located off the Pillars Lobby.

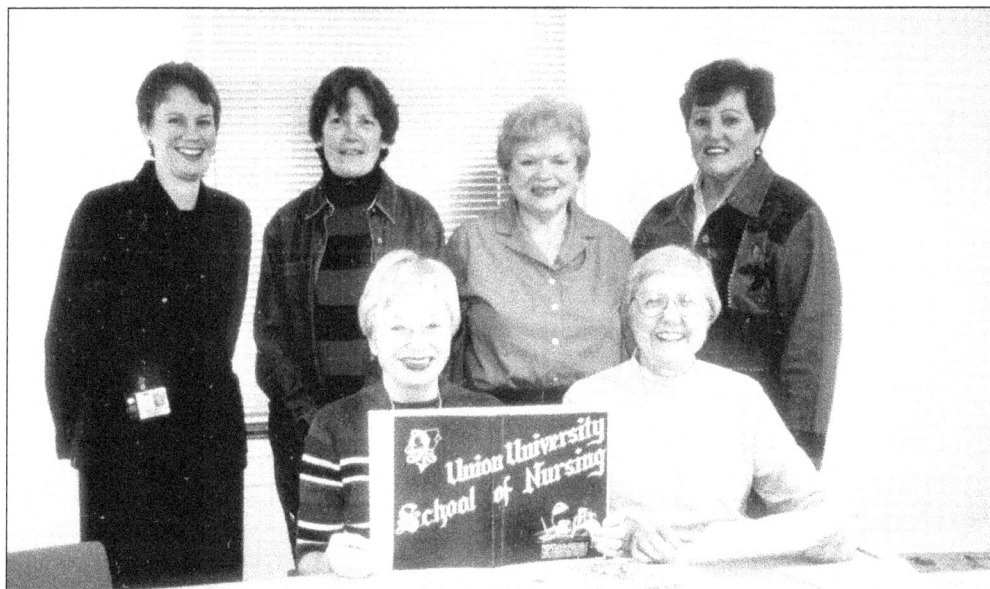

A Legacy of Nursing Work Session. Seated are Sandra Scudder (left) and Mary French. Standing are, from left to right, Connie Walsh, administrative director of annual programs for the Albany Medical Center Foundation; Elsie Whiting; Janet Gardner; and Paula Zenzen. This core group, with the help of hospital staff, alumni, and community members far and near, assisted in the completion of this publication.

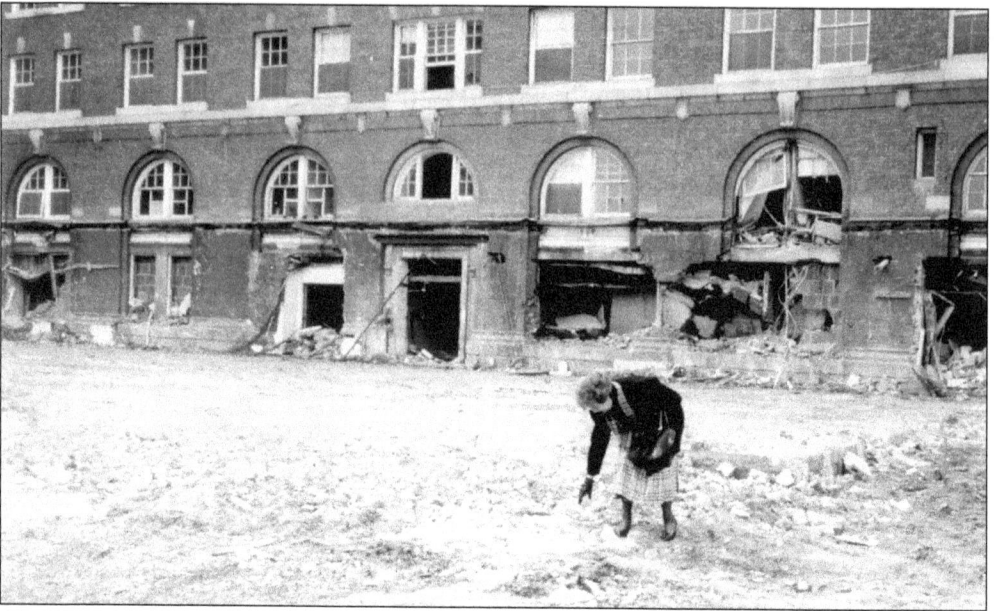

THE DEMOLITION HAS BEGUN. Audrey Woolsey searches for anything she might save from the rubble of the nurses' residence. Perhaps it was from this experience that the alumni's idea came of preserving some of the bricks and affixing a commemorative plaque.

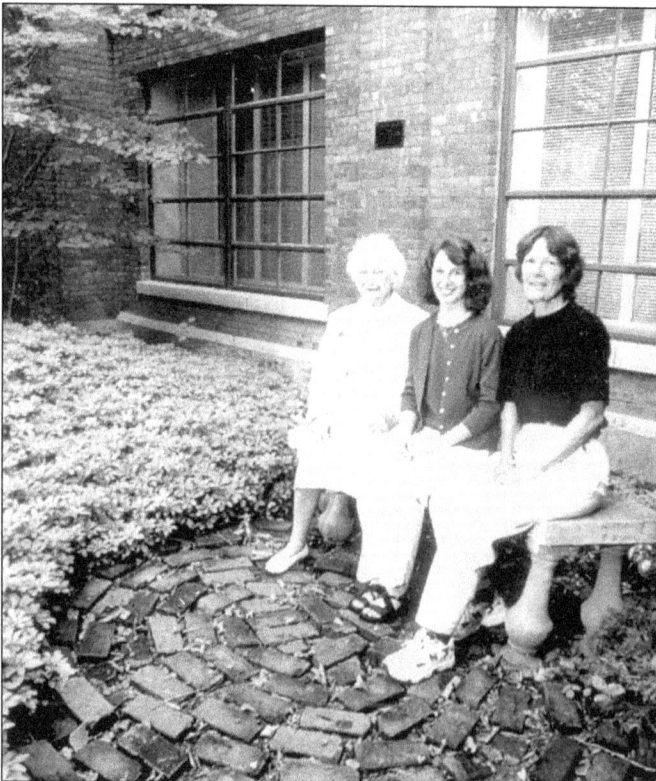

ADDITIONAL RESIDENCE BRICKS PRESERVED. Evelyn Sturdevan, volunteer extraordinaire at Albany Medical Center, decided that another place to preserve additional bricks from the nurses' residence was in the courtyard at the Albany Visitors Center at Quackenbush Square. The Alumni Association erected a plaque in 2002 denoting the placement and origin of the bricks. Seated are, from left to right, Evelyn Sturdevan; Kathy Quandt, director of operations at Albany Visitors Center; and Elsie Whiting.

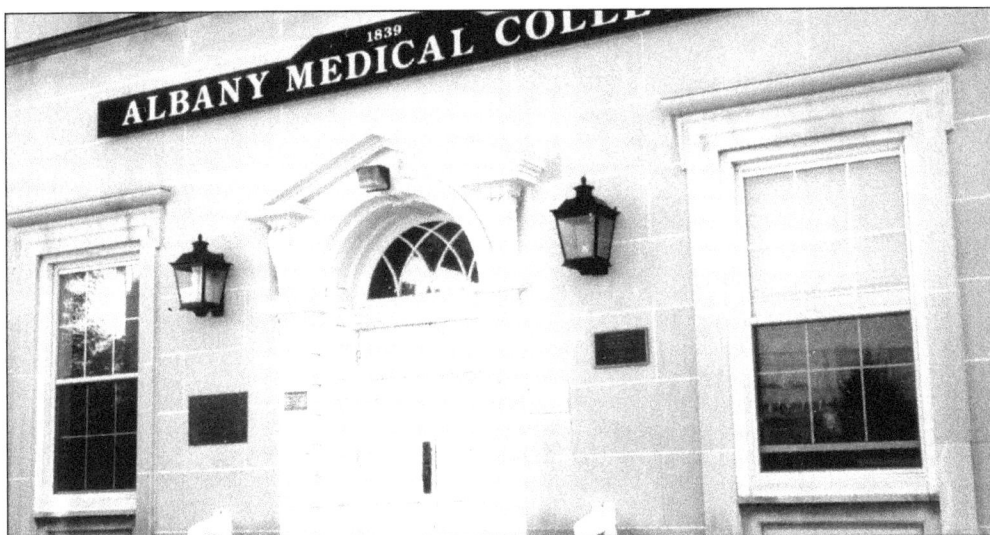

THE LANTERNS HAVE A NEW HOME. The lanterns mounted on either side of the entrance to Albany Medical College had previously lighted the Myrtle Avenue entrance to the nurses' residence, which was razed in 1988.

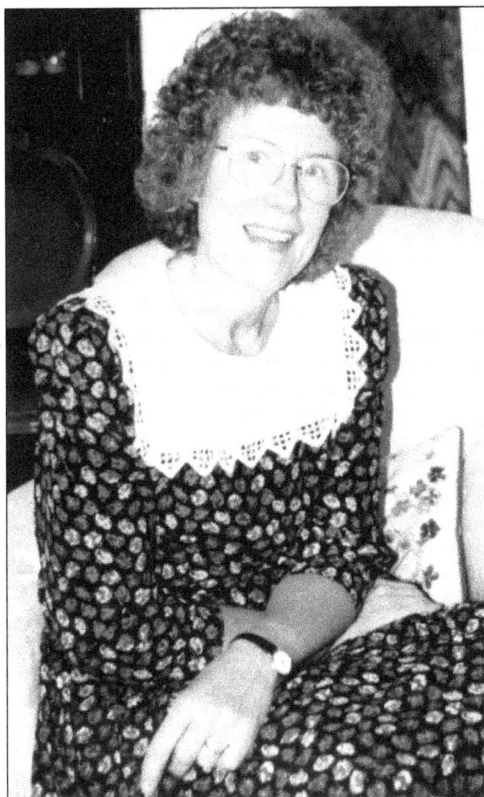

SUSAN ALLEN CLEMENTS, R.N., CLASS OF 1959, A MISSIONARY NURSE IN TANZANIA. After her graduation, Susan Allen went to England and completed a course in midwifery. Following her marriage, she and her husband became missionaries, and they have served in Tanzania since 1967. Clements became a midwifery tutor in 1988 at Koala Ndoto Hospital School of Nursing. This included classroom teaching and supervising students in the villages when they did their community fieldwork. Upon becoming qualified midwives, the students would return to their villages to help their own people.

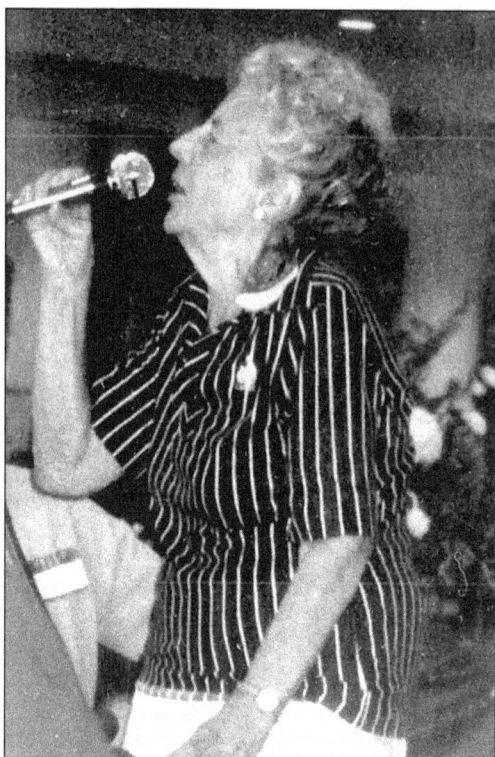

LOUISE RICE, R.N., CLASS OF 1932.
Celebrating 70 years since their graduation, the Class of 1932 had a telephone conference on May 18, 2002, following the alumni reunion. All seven living members of the class participated. At the reunion, Louise Rice closed the program by singing in a strong voice "May the Good Lord Bless and Keep You." Needless to say, there was not a dry eye in the place.

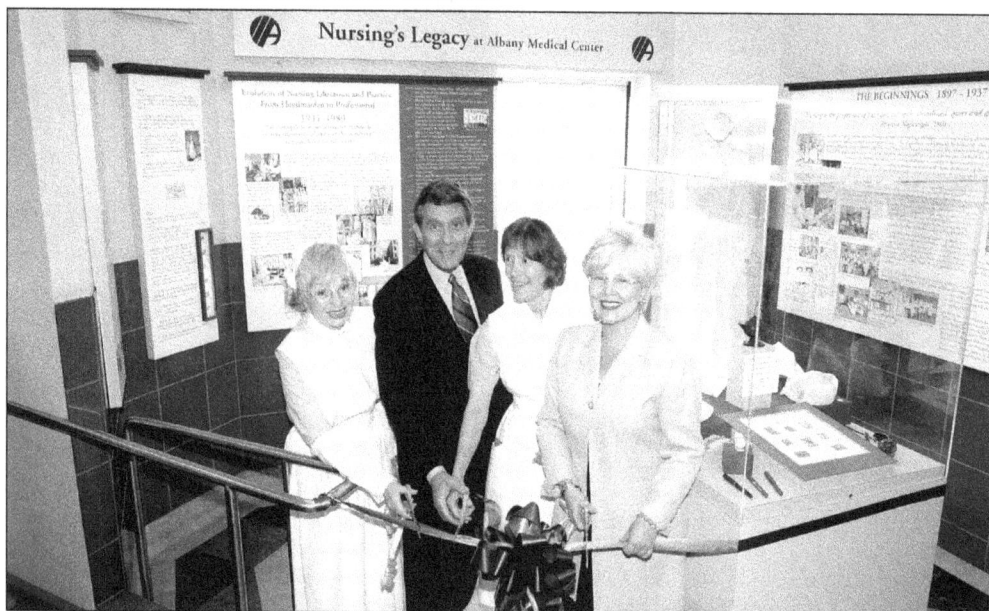

THE RIBBON CUTTING FOR A PERMANENT NURSING HISTORY EXHIBIT. From left to right are Sandra Scudder, director of AMCSN from 1987 to 1989; James J. Barba, president, chief executive officer, and chairman of the board of directors; Elsie Whiting, alumni president; and Mary Jo LaPosta, Ph.D., R.N., senior vice president and chief nursing officer (C.N.O.), cutting the ribbon for the exhibit *Nursing's Legacy at Albany Medical Center*, located off the Pillars Lobby. The ceremony took place during Nurse Recognition Week in May 2003.

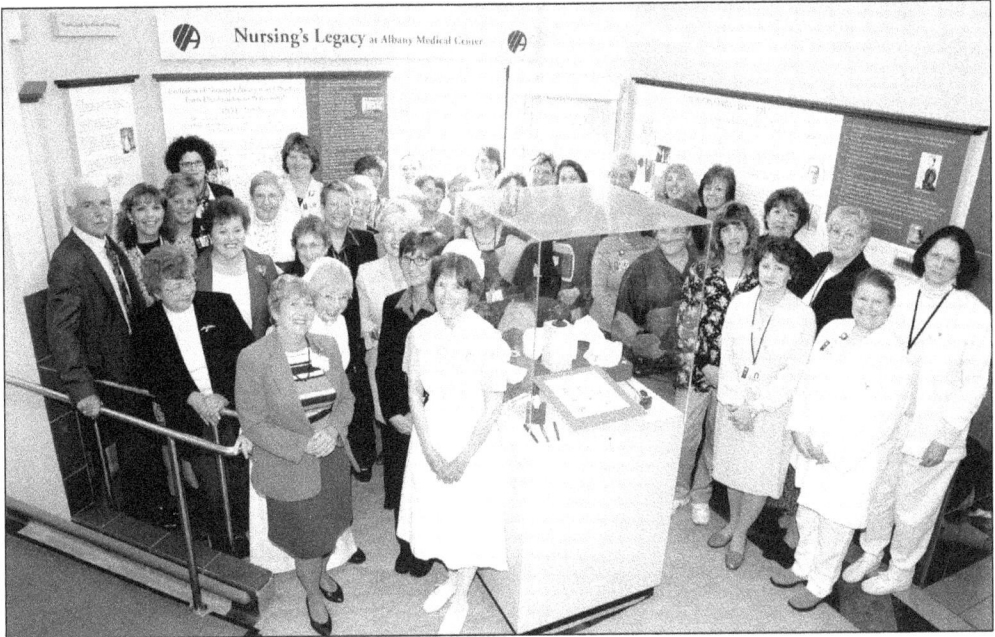

NURSES APPROVE THE DISPLAY. Nurse leaders, nursing school alumni, and nursing staff pose proudly in front of the nursing history exhibit near the Pillars Lobby. Dressed in the former student uniforms are Sandra Scudder in the AHTSN uniform (left) and Elsie Whiting in the UUSN uniform (right).

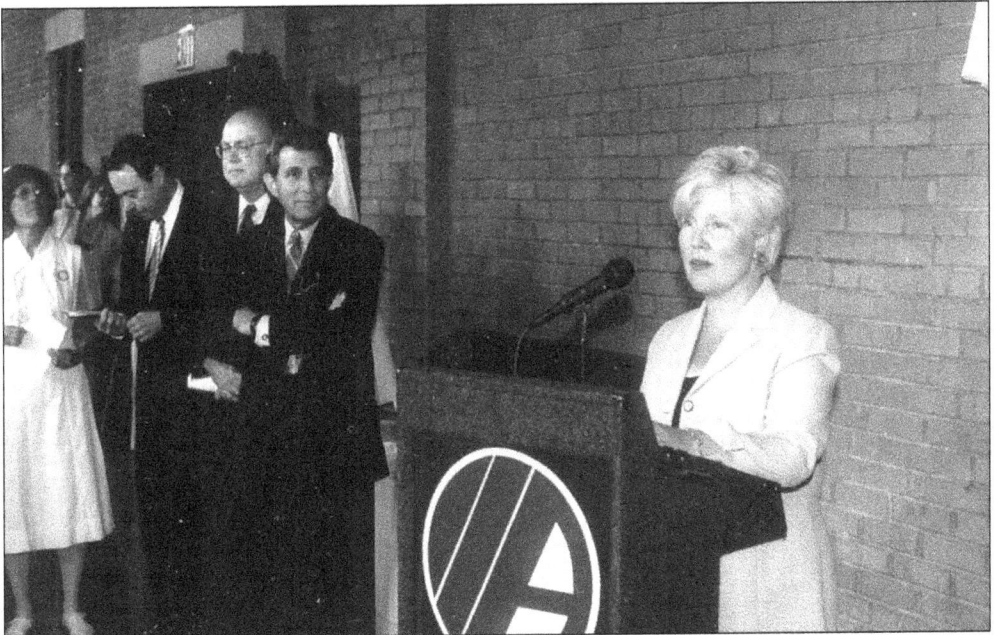

THE RECEPTION AT THE LAKE HOUSE IN WASHINGTON PARK. After the ribbon cutting for the nursing history exhibit, everyone gathered for a gala reception at the Lake House. Speakers included, from left to right, Elsie Whiting; Ron Canestrari, deputy majority leader of the New York State Assembly; Ray Sweeney, executive vice president of the Hospital Association of New York State; James J. Barba; and Mary Jo LaPosta.

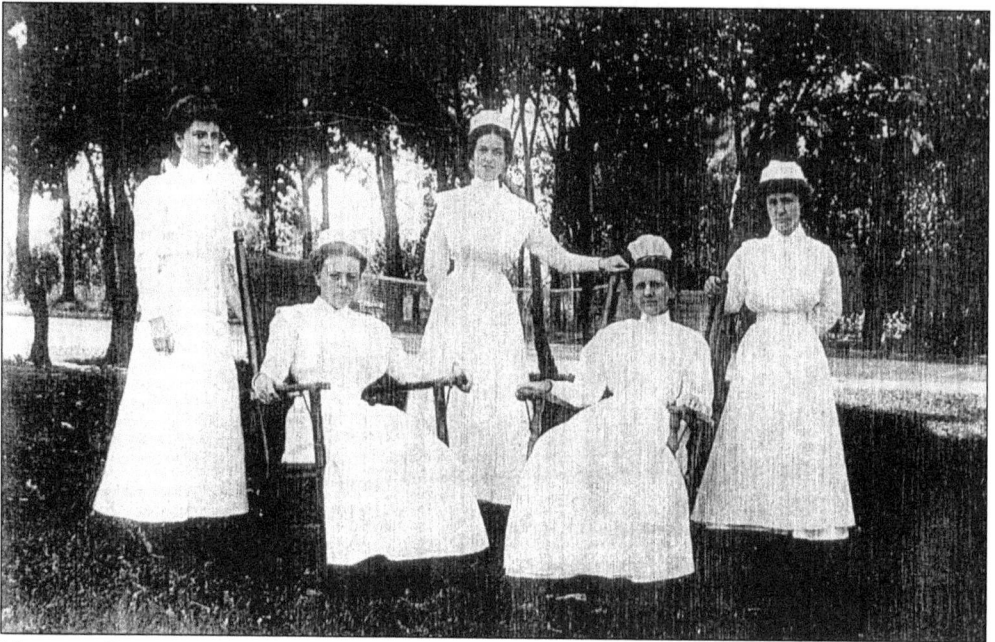

Nursing Supervisors. These nurses were in charge of all nursing at the hospital, including cleaning, in 1896. The person without a cap is a diet mistress. This was the attire for all official and professional functions. Contrast the attire of the 2003 nursing administrative staff.

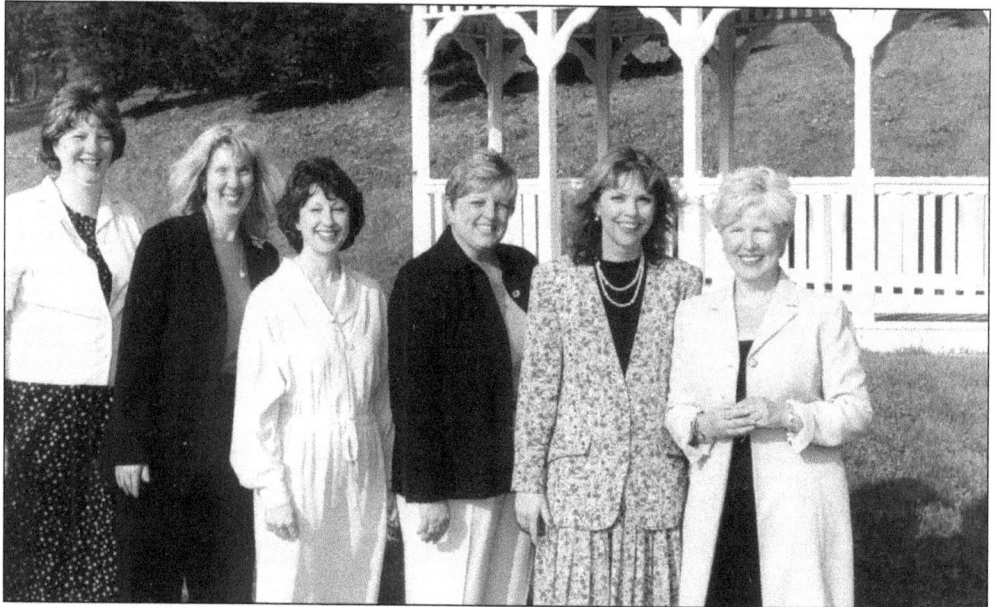

Mary Jo LaPosta, C.N.O., and Nursing Administrative Staff, 2003. From left to right are Karen Houston, M.S, R.N., director for quality and continuum of care; Lynne Longtin, M.S., R.N., patient care service director for heart, medical, surgical, and critical care services; Karen Clement-O'Brien, M.S., R.N., director of education development; Lin Lowden, M.S., R.N., patient care service director for women, children, and mental health services; Mary Ellen Plass, M.S., R.N., patient care service director for medical, surgical, and interventional services; and Mary Jo LaPosta, Ph.D., R.N.